Oculoplastic Surgery Atlas

Springer
New York
Berlin
Heidelberg
Barcelona
Hong Kong
London
Milan
Paris
Singapore
Tokyo

With Foreword by *Frank A. Nesi, MD, FAACS*
With Illustrations by *Timothy C. Hengst, CMI*
With Contributions by

Briggs E. Cook, MD
Oculoplastics Services
Department of Ophthalmology and Visual Sciences
University of Wisconsin–Madison
Ophthalmic Facial Plastic Surgery
Davis Duehr Dean Clinic
Madison, Wisconsin

Bradley N. Lemke, MD, FAACS
Clinical Professor of Ophthalmic Facial Plastic Surgery
Department of Ophthalmology and Visual Sciences
University of Wisconsin–Madison
Lemke Eye Plastic Surgery
Madison, Wisconsin

Mark J. Lucarelli, MD
Assistant Professor of Opthalmology
Oculoplastics Services
Department of Ophthalmology and Visual Sciences
University of Wisconsin–Madison
Madison, Wisconsin

John G. Rose, Jr., MD
Oculoplastics Services
Department of Ophthalmology and Visual Sciences
University of Wisconsin–Madison
Madison, Wisconsin

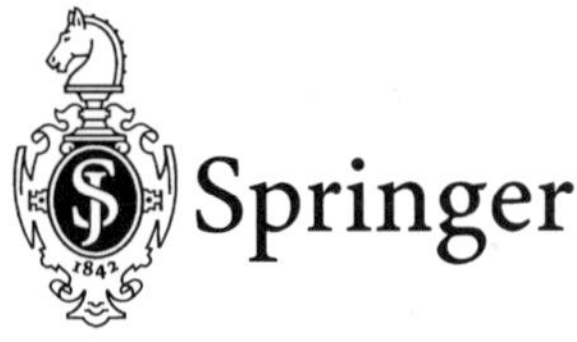

Springer

Oculoplastic Surgery Atlas
Eyelid Disorders

With 77 Illustrations

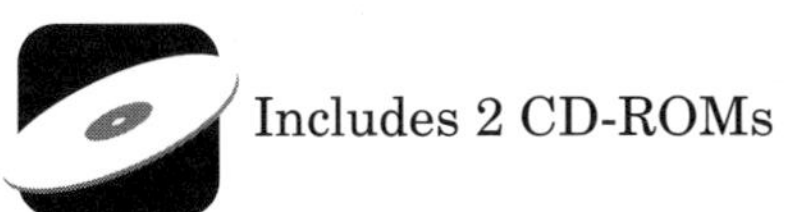 Includes 2 CD-ROMs

Geoffrey J. Gladstone, MD, FAACS
Assistant Clinical Professor of Ophthalmology and Otolaryngology, Wayne State University School of Medicine, Detroit, MI; Co-Director, Oculoplastic Surgery, Department of Ophthalmology, William Beaumont Hospital, Royal Oak, MI; Consultants in Ophthalmic and Facial Plastic Surgery, Southfield, MI, USA

Evan H. Black, MD, FAACS
Assistant Professor of Ophthalmology; Co-Director, Oculoplastic Surgery, Kresge Eye Institute, Wayne State University School of Medicine, Detroit, MI; Consultants in Ophthalmic and Facial Plastic Surgery, Southfield, MI, USA

Shoib Myint, DO, FAACS
Assistant Clinical Professor of Ophthalmology and Otolaryngology, Wayne State University School of Medicine, Detroit, MI; Co-Director, Oculoplastic Surgery, Department of Ophthalmology, William Beaumont Hospital, Royal Oak, MI; Consultants in Ophthalmic and Facial Plastic Surgery, Southfield, MI, USA

Brian G. Brazzo, MD, FAACS
Assistant Professor of Ophthalmology, Weill Medical College of Cornell University, New York, NY; Director, Oculoplastic Service, Department of Ophthalmology, Maimonides Medical Center, Brooklyn, NY; Assistant Attending Surgeon, Department of Ophthalmology, Manhattan Eye, Ear & Throat Hospital, New York, NY, USA

EDITOR EMERITUS
Frank A. Nesi, MD, FAACS
Assistant Clinical Professor of Ophthalmology and Otolaryngology; Co-Director, Oculoplastic Surgery, Kresge Eye Institute, Wayne State University School of Medicine, Detroit, MI; Director, Oculoplastic Surgery, Department of Ophthalmology, William Beaumont Hospital, Royal Oak, MI; Consultants in Ophthalmic and Facial Plastic Surgery, Southfield, MI, USA

Geoffrey J. Gladstone, MD, FAACS
Assistant Clinical Professor of Ophthalmology and
Otolaryngology, Wayne State University School of
Medicine, Detroit, MI 48202; Co-Director, Oculo-
plastic Surgery, Department of Ophthalmology,
William Beaumont Hospital, Royal Oak, MI
48073; Consultants in Ophthalmic and Facial
Plastic Surgery, Southfield, MI 48034, USA

Shoib Myint, DO, FAACS
Assistant Clinical Professor of Ophthalmology and
Otolaryngology, Wayne State University School of
Medicine, Detroit, MI 48202; Co-Director, Oculo-
plastic Surgery, Department of Ophthalmology,
William Beaumont Hospital, Royal Oak, MI
48073; Consultants in Ophthalmic and Facial
Plastic Surgery, Southfield, MI 48034, USA

Frank A. Nesi, MD, FAACS
Assistant Clinical Professor of Ophthalmology and
Otolaryngology; Co-Director, Oculoplastic Surgery,
Kresge Eye Institute, Wayne State University
School of Medicine, Detroit, MI 48202; Director,
Oculoplastic Surgery, Department of Ophthalmol-
ogy, William Beaumont Hospital, Royal Oak, MI
48073; Consultants in Ophthalmic and Facial
Plastic Surgery, Southfield, MI 48034, USA

Evan H. Black, MD, FAACS
Assistant Professor of Ophthalmology; Co-Director,
Oculoplastic Surgery, Kresge Eye Institute, Wayne
State University School of Medicine, Detroit, MI,
48202; Consultants in Ophthalmic and Facial Plastic
Surgery, Southfield, MI 48034, USA

Brian G. Brazzo, MD, FAACS
Assistant Professor of Ophthalmology, Weill Medical
College of Cornell University, New York, NY 14853;
Director, Oculoplastic Service, Department of Oph-
thalmology, Maimonides Medical Center, Brooklyn,
NY 11219; Assistant Attending Surgeon, Department
of Ophthalmology, Manhattan Eye, Ear & Throat
Hospital, New York, NY 10021, USA

Cover illustration: Timothy C. Hengst, CMI

Library of Congress Cataloging-in-Publication Data

Oculoplastic surgery atlas: eyelid disorders/editors, Geoffrey J. Gladstone...[et al.].
    p. ; cm.
    Includes bibliographical references and index.
    ISBN 0-387-95316-7 (h/c : alk. paper)
    1. Eyelids–Surgery–Atlases.   I. Title: Eyelid disorders.   II. Gladstone, Geoffrey J.
    [DNLM: 1. Eyelid Disease–surgery–Atlases.   2. Reconstructive Surgical
Procedures–Atlases.   WW 17 O212 2001]
RD119.5.E94 O285 2001
617.7'71059–dc21   2001041111

Printed on acid-free paper.

Production managed by Frank McGuckin; manufacturing supervised by Erica Bresler.
Typeset by Matrix Publishing Services, Inc., York, PA.
Printed and bound by Maple-Vail Book Manufacturing Group, York, PA.
Printed in the United States of America.

9 8 7 6 5 4 3 2 1

ISBN 0-387-95316-7   SPIN 10841539

Springer-Verlag New York Berlin Heidelberg
A member of BertelsmannSpringer Science+Business Media GmbH

There is no greater joy in medicine than to pass on knowledge. The benefits are innumerable. Patients receive better care, the physician practices a higher quality of medicine, and the field of medicine achieves a more advanced state by the synthesis of knowledge from many sources.

The teacher's benefits are less obvious, but just as meaningful and rewarding. Seeing residents or practicing physicians broaden their knowledge or perfect a new surgical technique provides a wonderful sense of accomplishment. It is also a way to repay those who have selflessly given their knowledge in the past.

This book is dedicated to those who seek knowledge. It is hoped that in some small way this CD-ROM and book set will improve your practice of medicine and simplify the application of appropriate oculofacial surgical procedures.

Geoffrey J. Gladstone, MD, FAACS

FOREWORD

The desire to teach and the fulfillment attained from teaching have again prompted us to produce a work that we hope will be both useful and enlightening to our readers.

The field of oculoplastic surgery has grown and evolved to include all aspects of eyelid and facial plastic surgery. Our literature must now reflect the advancements and direction of our field. Knowledge of anatomy, the basis of all surgery and the root of surgical principles and techniques, is the basis of our ability to deliver the highest-quality care to our patients.

We have therefore combined text and diagrams, and supplemented them with CD-ROM digital video technology to provide to those who wish to perform this surgery the best possible instruction and preparation. We hope that our attempts to accomplish this will be rewarded by the use of our material by our colleagues and the acknowledgment of our unique and logical progression in the field of eyelid and facial plastic surgery. Future volumes in this series will cover other aspects of eyelid, lacrimal, facial, and orbital surgery.

Frank A. Nesi, MD, FAACS

PREFACE

This will be the first text to closely coordinate high quality digital video footage of surgical procedures with a surgical atlas and text. The test will thoroughly cover patient evaluation and decision making for each procedure. This should allow the reader to choose the proper operation. The text will have a detailed description of the surgical procedure keyed to limited number diagrams. The description of the procedure follows the digital video footage on a separate CD-ROM.

The book is intended for ophthalmologists, ophthalmic plastic surgeons, ENT, general plastic surgeons and others wanting a better knowledge of eyelid surgery. It is geared at the beginner/intermediate level and includes only practical, immediately useful techniques. It is limited in scope to keep it practical and quickly producible.

Although many texts and surgical atlases exist, this will be the first with easily accessible digital footage of *every* procedure. This will be tightly edited footage exactly and completely showing each procedure. It will provide a *unique* learning experience for the reader as well as allowing Springer-Verlag to be the first to market this type of multimedia presentation.

More and more general ophthalmologist, ENT, and plastic surgeons are interested in eyelid surgery. This text will offer them a learning experience not obtainable elsewhere.

One or two more volumes are possible once the appeal of this format is demonstrated:

Volume II—Orbit, Trauma and Lacrimal Disorders
Volume III—Cosmetic Eyelid and Facial Surgery

Geoffrey J. Gladstone, MD, FAACS

ACKNOWLEDGMENTS

Bringing a book project to fruition is always a complicated process involving many people. It is through their dedication, professionalism, and team effort that it all comes together.

Timothy C. Hengst, CMI, our medical illustrator, deserves special recognition for the quality of his work; his illustrations clarify the text in a way that only visual images can. The tremendous ease with which we communicated digitally during the illustration process is particularly appreciated.

Laurel Craven, our executive editor, and the rest of the people at Springer-Verlag New York, Inc., have been kind, patient, and helpful. Their suggestions and directions have been instrumental in producing a unique and gratifying final product.

Our fellow, Dr. César Sierra, acquired an unexpected skill at the beginning of his training. In addition to his more medically related skills, he has become the best videographer we have. The quality of the videos start with his excellent photographic work.

Drs. Rose, Jr., Lucarelli, Cook, and Lemke contributed a concise, but comprehensive overview of clinically relevant eyelid anatomy. As always, anatomy is the basis for understanding the etiology of surgical problems and provides the guideposts for surgical corrections. The high caliber of our colleagues' work gives the reader an essential starting point in understanding and utilizing the techniques presented in this book.

Geoffrey J. Gladstone, MD, FAACS

CONTENTS

1

SURGICAL ANATOMY OF THE EYELID

- John G. Rose, Jr., MD
- Mark J. Lucarelli, MD
- Briggs E. Cook, MD
- Bradley N. Lemke, MD, FAACS

*Department of Ophthalmology and Visual Sciences,
University of Wisconsin–Madison, Madison, Wisconsin*

Proper diagnosis and management of eyelid disorders, both functional and cosmetic, hinge upon a thorough understanding of the location of critical eyelid structures and the anatomic relationships between them. Accurate intraoperative identification of anatomy is fundamental in performing eyelid surgery and preventing complications.

EYEBROW

As an important source of support for the eyelids and a major determinant in facial expression, the eyebrows should be included in any evaluation of eyelid dysfunction. Eyebrow position strongly influences eyelid position and architecture, and many cases of upper eyelid ptosis and apparent dermatochalasis are, in fact, a consequence of eyebrow ptosis. Similarly, frontalis muscle recruitment can mask significant blepharoptosis. In these situations, addressing only the lids may lead to an inadequate or undesirable surgical result.

The ideal contour of the eyebrows (Figure 1-1) is highly debated and varies according to age and gender. The female medial brow generally begins superior, or slightly superonasal, to the medial canthus; the lateral brow ends superotemporal to the lateral canthus, at the end of a line extending from the most lateral extent of the ala of the nose through the lateral canthus.[1] The medial and lateral ends of the brow are typically at the same vertical level, although the lateral brow may be slightly higher. The apex should lie above the region between the lateral limbus and the lateral canthus.[2] The male eyebrow generally rides lower and flatter than that of the female.[3]

Eyebrow contour and position are influenced by five principal muscles: frontalis, orbicularis, corrugator, procerus, and depressor supercilii. Contraction of the frontalis elevates the eyebrows, while contraction of the orbicularis depresses them. The corrugator depresses the medial eyebrows toward the midline and forms the vertical furrows in the glabella. The procerus depresses the glabella and forms horizontal wrinkles across the dorsum of the nose. The depressor supercilii also depresses the eyebrows medially, contributing to the formation of oblique glabellar wrinkles.

Beneath the eyebrow lies the eyebrow fat pad, which supports the eyebrow over the supraorbital ridge. Dense, fibrous attachments anchor the eyebrow to the supraorbital ridge. Because the ridge underlies only the medial one-third to one-half of the eyebrow, the lateral eyebrow lacks the same degree of underlying support. This has been proposed as an explanation for the fact that the lateral eyebrow often droops more than the medial eyebrow with age.[4]

EYELID TOPOGRAPHY

Eyelid topography (Figure 1-1) is influenced by age, race, ethnicity, and surrounding facial anatomy, particularly that of the eyebrow. In most individuals, the lateral canthus sits 2 mm higher than the medial canthus, with slightly greater elevation in individuals of Asian descent. The adult interpalpebral distance measures 28–30 mm horizontally and 9–12 mm at its greatest vertical extent centrally. The upper eyelid margin rests approximately 1–2 mm below the superior limbus. The lower eyelid margin rests at the inferior limbus. Laxity of the canthal ligaments not only causes poor apposition of the eyelids to the globe, but also changes the contour of the interpalpebral

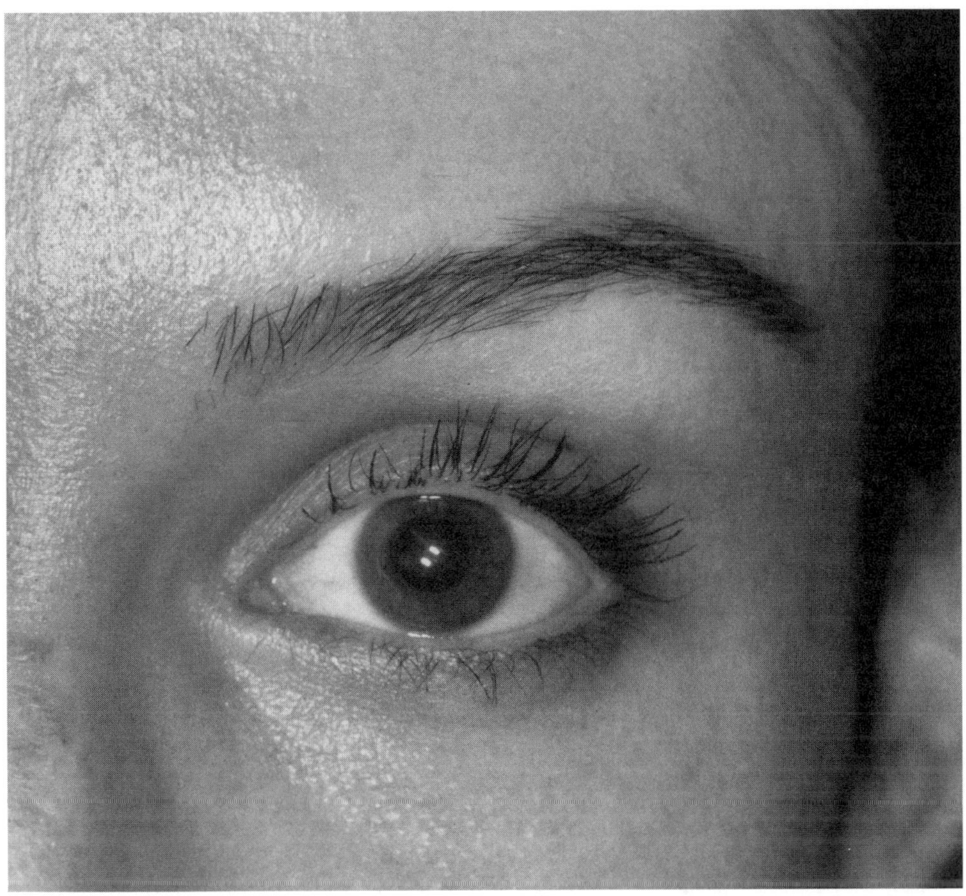

FIGURE 1-1. Topographic eyelid and eyebrow anatomy in the adult female. The eyebrow is gently arched, with the highest point above the temporal limbus. The highest point of the upper eyelid is slightly nasal to the center of the pupil, while the lower eyelid margin lies at the inferior limbus.

fissure. The upper eyelid is gently curved, with the highest point nasal to the center of the pupil.[5,6]

The upper eyelid crease is an important surgical landmark, as it is often an incision site. The crease is formed by the superficial insertions of the levator aponeurosis[7] and should generally be re-formed if these attachments are disturbed.[8] It rides parallel to the lid margin and lies 8–11 mm above the eyelid margin in women and 7–8 mm above in men.[6] In people of European ancestry, the septum-levator insertion occurs 2–5 mm superior to the upper edge of the tarsus.[9] In Asians, the orbital septum inserts low on the levator aponeurosis,[9] below the superior tarsal border,[10] yielding a low or poorly defined lid crease.[11] This is an important point to keep in mind when operating on Asian eyelids.

The lower eyelid crease is less prominent. It begins medially 4–5 mm below the lower eyelid margin. It slopes inferiorly as it proceeds laterally. It is formed by fibers that extend anteriorly from the capsulopalpebral fascia into the subcutaneous tissues.[12]

EYELID SKIN AND MARGIN

The eyelid skin is the thinnest in the body, mainly owing to its attenuated dermis. Eyelid incisions therefore heal rapidly. The thinness of the skin also helps to keep scarring to a minimum. As it crosses over the orbital rim, the eyelid skin abruptly thickens.

The surface of the eyelid margin contains numerous important anatomical landmarks (Figure 1-2) for eyelid surgery. The upper eyelid margin has approximately 100 eyelashes, while the lower has about 50. Several sebaceous Zeiss glands empty into each lash follicle, while Moll sweat glands are located between follicles. Posterior to the lash line on the eyelid margin is the easily noticeable line of meibomian glands, which emanate from the edge of the tarsus. Between the lash line and the meibomian line lies a faint gray line, which is more pronounced in younger individuals. This represents the edge of the muscle of Riolan. The gray line serves as an important surgical landmark, separating the eyelid vertically into the anterior lamella—skin and orbicularis—and posterior lamella: tarsus, retractors, and conjunctiva.[13]

EYELID CONNECTIVE TISSUE

Orbital Septum

The orbital septum (Figure 1-2) is the boundary between the eyelids and orbit. It is commonly encountered during eyelid surgery and is easily identified by tugging inferiorly on it to confirm its strong attachment to the orbital rim. The orbital septum is a multilamellar layer of dense connective tissue that lines the orbit and terminates by fusing at the periosteum of the orbital rim. This termination forms the arcus marginalis.[9] Laterally, the septum inserts anteriorly onto

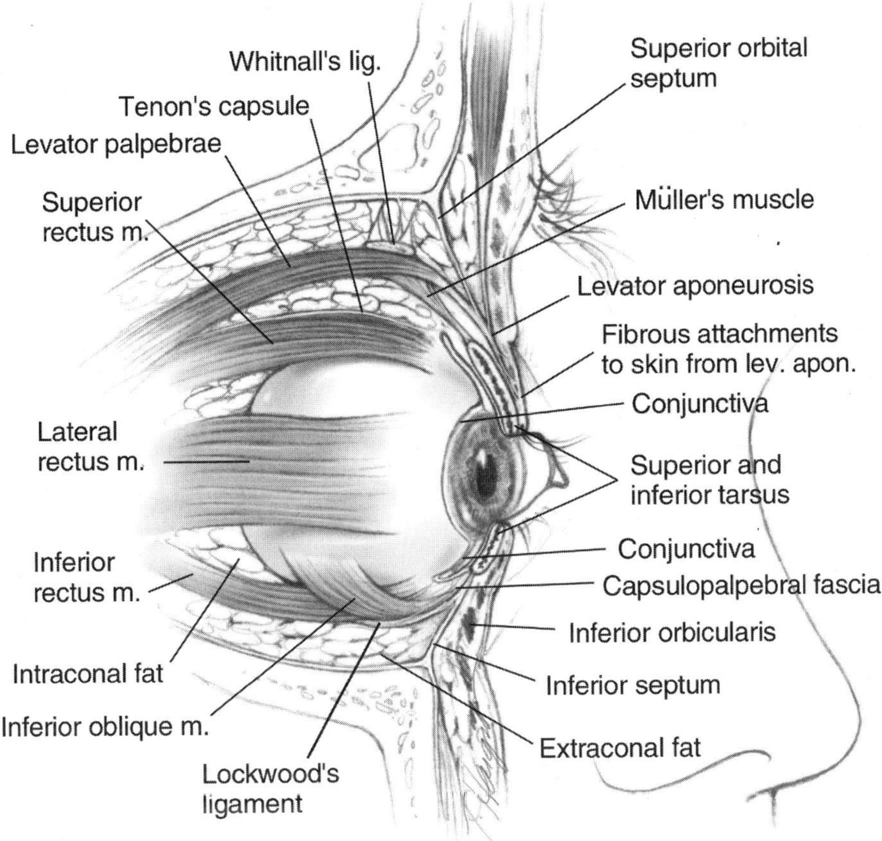

FIGURE 1-2. Parasagittal section of the orbit, showing eyelid structures.

the lateral canthal ligament and posteriorly on Whitnall's tubercle on the lateral orbital rim. Medially, the septum splits and inserts to both the posterior and anterior lacrimal crest. Multiple fibrous attachments emanate from the orbital septum, anchoring it anteriorly to the orbicularis muscle.[14] The preaponeurotic fat lies immediately posterior to the orbital septum. In the lower eyelid, the orbital septum fuses with the capsulopalpebral fascia 5 mm inferior to the lower border of the tarsus.[12]

The strength of the orbital septum varies among individuals, as well as with age. Age often results in attenuation of the septum, resulting in anterior prolapse of orbital fat.[6]

The orbital septum serves as a barrier to infection. Eyelid infection that remains anterior to the septum and is therefore confined from the orbit by the septum is termed preseptal cellulitis. When infection crosses an intact or violated septum, orbital cellulitis results, a vision-threatening, and, in some cases, life-threatening condition.

Tarsal Plates

The tarsal plates (Figure 1-2) provide rigidity to the eyelids. They are composed of dense, fibrous connective tissue. The upper tarsus measures 10–12 mm vertically, while the lower measures 3–5 mm.[15] The tarsal borders adjacent to the lid margin are straight, while the opposite edges have a convex curvature. The posterior edge of the tarsus is firmly attached to the palpebral conjunctiva, which extends to the eyelid margin and terminates at the gray line.

Within the tarsus lie branched, acinar, sebaceous glands with long central ducts. Known as the meibomian glands, they open at the eyelid margin, just posterior to the gray line, and secrete the oily layer of the tear film. There are about 25 in the upper eyelid and about 20 in the lower.[9] Inflammation of these glands, known as meibomitis, may, over a long term, result in distichiasis,[16] or abnormal hair follicles that, unlike the normal eyelashes, curve inward toward the globe, resulting in discomfort and possibly corneal abrasion. A common treatment for distichiasis, electrohyfrecation, may cause focal necrosis of the tarsus, resulting in notching at the eyelid margin.[6] Similarly, excessive cryotherapy for distichiasis can cause a wider-than-planned area of lash loss and scarring.

Canthal Ligaments

Emanating from the medial and lateral borders of the tarsi and anchoring them to the orbital rim are the canthal ligaments. These are formed by a fusion of the upper and lower crura, the thickened extensions of the margins of the upper and lower tarsi, respectively. These support not only the tarsi, but also the orbicularis. The medial canthal ligament splits into three arms: anterior, posterior, and superior. The anterior arm attaches to the maxillary bone, anterior to the lacrimal crest. The posterior arm attaches to the posterior lacrimal crest.[17,18] The superior arm inserts onto the orbital process of the frontal bone.[19] The lateral canthal ligament inserts 1.5 mm inside the lateral orbital rim at Whitnall's tubercle, on the zygomatic bone.[20] In lower eyelid tightening procedures, which usually involve surgical manipulation of the lateral aspect of the lower tarsus and the lateral canthal ligament, the posterior direction and insertion of the lateral canthal ligament must be preserved. Laxity of the canthal ligaments can cause ectropion, as well as a cosmetically apparent shortening of the horizontal palpebral fissure.[21]

Whitnall's Ligament and Levator Aponeurosis

An important support for the upper eyelid is Whitnall's ligament. Its role has been debated[14]; it may serve as a fulcrum-like check ligament for the levator or as a swinging suspender providing vertical support for the upper eyelid.[20,22] Despite this debate, it is understood that Whitnall's ligament suspends the lacrimal gland, superior oblique ligament, levator muscle (with the primary support for the levator coming from the globe), and Tenon's capsule. Whitnall's ligament is a transverse fibrous condensation that inserts medially inside the superomedial orbital rim on the frontal bone at the trochlea and laterally inside the superolateral orbital rim, near the frontozygomatic suture, where it fuses with fibers of the lacrimal gland capsule. It encircles the levator complex[23] at the level of the junction of the levator muscle and the fibrous levator aponeurosis. The aponeurosis extends another 14–20 mm inferior to Whitnall's ligament to insert on the lower third of the anterior face of the upper tarsus. Dehiscence of the levator aponeurosis is responsible for many cases of involutional ptosis, and when encountered during ptosis repair, it can be identified as a band of pearly, white tissue that retracts on attempted upgaze.

EYELID MUSCULATURE

Orbicularis Oculi, Muscle of Riolan, and Horner's Muscle

The orbicularis oculi muscle (Figure 1-2) surrounds the anterior orbit and can be divided into three components: pretarsal, preseptal, and orbital.[24] The pretarsal orbicularis originates from the anterior and posterior arms of the medial canthal ligament. It is firmly adherent to the anterior face of the tarsus and to the levator aponeurosis. Medially, the pretarsal orbicularis divides into a superficial head, which surrounds the canaliculi, and a deep head, which inserts on the posterior lacrimal crest and lacrimal fascia. These insertions allow the pretarsal orbicularis to play an important role in the lacrimal pump mechanism. The preseptal orbicularis originates from the upper and lower margins of the medial canthal ligament and inserts lateral to the orbital rim on the zygoma. It overlies the orbital septum and orbital rim, and it is separated from the septum by a fibrofatty layer, the postorbicularis fascia.[6] This layer is an important dissection plane in anterior eyelid tightening procedures. The orbital orbicularis originates from the maxillary and frontal bones, as well as from the medial canthal ligament; it overrides the orbital rims and inserts at the same location as the preseptal orbicularis. These latter two portions of the orbicularis are responsible for forced eyelid closure.

Two important components of the orbicularis are the muscle of Riolan and Horner's muscle. The muscle of Riolan is a small segment of the orbicularis that is separated from the pretarsal orbicularis by the eyelash follicles. It corresponds to the gray line seen at the eyelid margin.[13] The deep pretarsal head of the orbicularis is known as Horner's muscle. Contraction of this muscle pulls the eyelids medially and posteriorly. In so doing, Horner's muscle compresses the canaliculi and lacrimal ampullae, pushing tears toward the lacrimal sac.[25] This mechanism, known as the lacrimal pump,[26] can therefore be compromised by weakening or laxity of the eyelids, resulting in epiphora.[27]

Levator Palpebrae Superioris

The main retractor of the upper eyelid is the levator palpebrae superioris (Figure 1-2). It originates at the annulus of Zinn in the orbital apex and courses anteriorly through the superior orbit, along the superior aspect of the superior rectus muscle. As it approaches the upper eyelid, the levator is encircled by Whitnall's ligament.[23] At this point, the levator muscle transitions into the fibrous levator aponeurosis, which courses inferiorly for another 14–20 mm, to attach to the inferior third of the anterior surface of the tarsus. Also at the level of Whitnall's ligament, the levator sends off lateral and medial horns. The lateral horn attaches to the zygomatic bone. The medial horn fuses with the posterior arm of the medial canthal ligament and inserts on the posterior lacrimal crest. The lateral and medial horns help ensure that the upper eyelid maintains a curvature that keeps it apposed to the globe during opening.[5] The levator aponeurosis sends fibers anteriorly through the septum and orbicularis to the skin; these insertions form the upper eyelid crease.[7]

Aging affects both the levator muscle and the aponeurosis. Age-related thinning and dehiscence of the aponeurosis from the tarsus is a common cause of involutional ptosis.[28,29] In addition, the muscle belly can become infiltrated with fat and connective tissue.[6]

Müller's Muscle

Underlying the levator aponeurosis, and attached to it via loose connective tissue, is Müller's muscle, which is sympathetically innervated and composed of smooth muscle fibers. It originates from the undersurface of the levator and courses inferiorly for approximately 15 mm to insert on the superior edge of the tarsus in the upper eyelid. A lateral extension of Müller's muscle divides the lacrimal gland into its two lobes.[30] It is generally accepted that Müller's muscle is a secondary transmitter of lift to the upper eyelid, as evidenced by the 2–3 mm ptosis seen either in sympathetic denervation syndromes, such as Horner's syndrome, or in the normal fatigue-related decrease in sympathetic tone. One group has suggested that Müller's muscle may serve as a primary transmitter of levator muscle tone to the tarsal plate.[31]

Lower Eyelid Retractors

Less defined than their counterparts that elevate the upper eyelid, the lower eyelid retractors—the capsulopalpebral fascia and inferior tarsal muscle—are palpebral extensions of the inferior rectus muscle. The inferior rectus muscle, through these lower eyelid retractors, is responsible for the full extent of depression of the lower eyelid during downgaze.[6] A fibrous extension of the inferior rectus muscle, the capsulopalpebral head of the inferior rectus wraps around the inferior oblique muscle, at which point the capsulopalpebral head splits into superior and inferior divisions. The inferior division, which is the capsulopalpebral fascia, then rejoins the superior division, the inferior tarsal muscle,[12] which, like Müller's muscle, is composed of smooth muscle fibers. These two layers are not generally distinct during surgical dissection.

The lower eyelid retractors have three insertions. Posteriorly, the retractors insert on Tenon's fascia. Centrally, the inferior tarsal muscle fibers terminate a few millimeters inferior to the tarsus,[12] and a fibrous continuation attaches to the inferior border of the tarsus. Anteriorly, the capsulopalpebral fascia fuses with the orbital septum 4 mm inferior to the tarsus. Fibers continue through the septum and attach to the subcutaneous tissue, forming the lower eyelid crease.[5]

EYELID FAT PADS

The eyelid fat pads (Figure 1-2) play an important role in the appearance and contour of the eyelids. In the youthful face, eyelid fat imparts a fullness and smoothness to the upper and lower eyelids. With age, atrophy of eyelid fat can cause the eyelids to sink posteriorly, resulting in involutional enophthalmos and a lid crease displaced away from the lid margin.[21] In addition, weakening of the orbital septum can allow anterior prolapse of the eyelid fat, resulting in a puffy appearance known as steatoblepharon.[3,5]

The upper eyelid contains two fat pads, which are located posterior to the orbital septum and immediately anterior to the levator muscle and aponeurosis. This anatomical relationship is convenient for the eyelid surgeon who wishes to combine levator aponeurosis repair with blepharoplasty and/or fat pad excision. This region of the upper eyelid is divided into three fibrous compartments. The medial and central compartments contain the two fat pads, while the lateral compartment contains the lacrimal gland.[32] Care must be taken not to confuse the lacrimal gland with eyelid fat in the upper eyelid. The lacrimal gland sits lateral to the two upper eyelid fat pads, and in contrast to the glistening, yellow, loose-appearing fat, it appears pink and firm.

The lower eyelid contains three fat pads, which are enclosed in three fibrous compartments: medial, central, and lateral. The inferior oblique muscle courses between the medial and central compartments in the lower eyelid, and care must be taken not to damage it in lower eyelid fat excision. The lower eyelid fat pads are contiguous with posterior orbital fat, as is the medial fat pad in the upper eyelid; care must therefore be taken not to cause excessive traction on the lower fat pads intraoperatively, as orbital hemorrhage may result in the intra- or postoperative period.

EYELID VASCULATURE

Arteries

The eyelids are highly vascularized, and knowledge of vascular anatomy is critical to avoiding complications during eyelid surgery. Eyelid blood supply (Figure 1-3) arises from both the external and internal carotid arteries. The external carotid artery gives rise to the facial artery, the superficial temporal artery and the infraorbital ar-

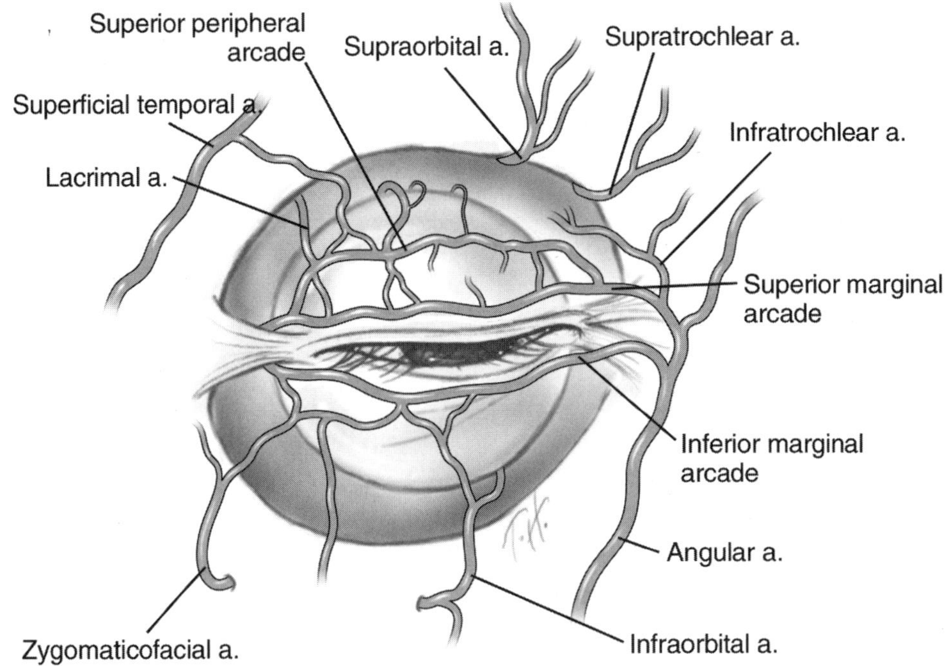

FIGURE 1-3. Arterial blood supply to the eyelids.

tery. As it courses across the face diagonally toward the nasolabial folds, the facial artery becomes the angular artery, which lies directly beneath the orbicularis and feeds the vascular arcades of the eyelids at the medial canthus. The internal carotid artery gives rise to the ophthalmic artery, which in turn terminates as the lacrimal, frontal, supraorbital and supratrochlear, and nasal arteries. Anastomoses between the angular, lacrimal, and supratrochlear arteries form the superior marginal arcade and superior peripheral arcade in the upper eyelid. The angular artery anastomoses in the lower eyelid with the infraorbital and zygomaticofacial arteries to form the inferior marginal arcade. A poorly developed inferior peripheral arcade may be present in some individuals.[5,6]

In the upper and lower eyelids, the marginal arcades lie just anterior to the tarsi, 2–4 mm from the eyelid margin. Also in the upper eyelid, the superior peripheral arcade lies just anterior to Müller's muscle, superior to the tarsus. This arcade not only serves the upper part of the upper eyelid, but also supplies the superior conjunctival fornix and communicates with the anterior ciliary vessels near the limbus. Dissection in the plane of Müller's muscle can cause hemorrhage from this arcade.[6]

Veins

The facial vein is the principal venous drainage source for the eyelids. It courses superficial and lateral to the facial artery. It begins near the medial canthus as the angular vein and anastomoses with the superior ophthalmic vein via the supraorbital vein.

Lymphatics

Lymphatic drainage of the medial portions of the eyelids and conjunctiva follows the course of the facial vein to the submandibular nodes. Lateral portions of the eyelid and conjunctiva drain into the preauricular lymph nodes.

EYELID INNERVATION

Sensory Innervation

The eyelids are innervated by the facial nerve (cranial nerve VII), the oculomotor nerve (cranial nerve III), the trigeminal nerve (cranial nerve V) and sympathetic fibers from the superior cervical ganglion. Sensory innervation to the upper eyelid is provided by the ophthalmic division of the trigeminal nerve (cranial nerve V_1), which has three branches—lacrimal, frontal, and nasociliary—all of which enter the orbit via the superior orbital fissure. The lacrimal nerve supplies the lacrimal gland conjunctiva and lateral upper eyelid, and it sends off a branch that anastomoses with the zygomaticotemporal nerve. The frontal nerve courses anteriorly between the periorbita and levator, dividing into the supraorbital and supratrochlear nerves. The supratrochlear nerve innervates the medial upper eyelid and forehead, while the two divisions of the supraorbital nerve innervates most of the remainder of the forehead. A superficial division passes anterior to the frontalis muscle to innervate the forehead skin, and a deep division that passes laterally anterior to the pericranium and supplies the frontoparietal scalp.[33] The nasociliary branch gives rise to the posterior and anterior ethmoidal nerves, two or three long ciliary nerves to the globe, a sensory root to the ciliary ganglion, and a sensory root to the infratrochlear nerve.[6]

Sensory innervation to the lower eyelid is provided by the maxillary branch of the trigeminal nerve (cranial nerve V_2). The zygomatic branch from V_3 divides into the zygomaticofacial and zygomaticotemporal nerves. The zygomaticofacial nerve courses along the inferolateral orbit, passes through the zygomaticofacial foramen, and supplies the skin of the cheek. The zygomaticotemporal nerve exits the orbit into the temporal fossa, innervating the lateral forehead. The infraorbital nerve, a continuation of V_2, exits via the infraorbital foramen, yielding several terminal branches—the inferior palpebral, lateral nasal, and superior labial nerves—which supply the skin and conjunctiva of the lower eyelid, the skin and septum of the nose, and the skin and mucosa of the upper lip, respectively.[6]

Motor Innervation

Motor innervation to the levator comes from the superior division of the oculomotor nerve (cranial nerve III). This division courses within the muscle cone of the orbit, entering the superior rectus from its inferior aspect, 15 mm from the orbital apex. At this point, it also sends off terminal fibers, which pass around or through the medial aspect of the superior rectus to innervate the levator.

The frontal and orbicularis muscles are innervated by divisions of the facial nerve (Figure 1-4). After originating at its nucleus in the

FIGURE 1-4. Anatomy of the facial nerve (cranial nerve VII).

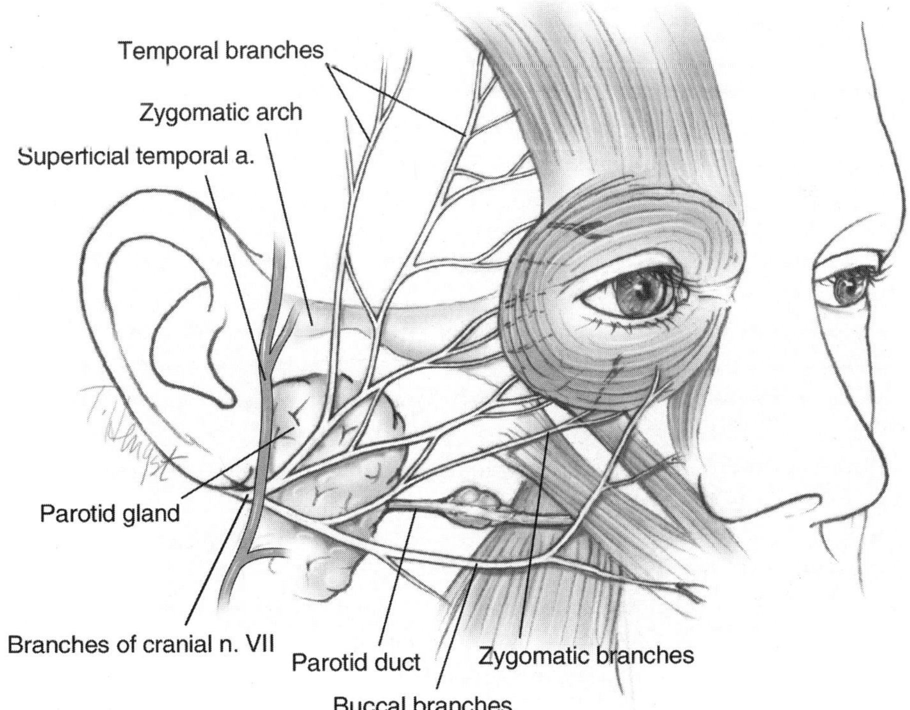

pons, the facial nerve leaves the facial canal via the stylomastoid foramen. It then passes through the parotid gland and gives rise to several divisions: temporal, zygomatic, buccal, mandibular, and cervical nerves. The temporal branch innervates the frontalis muscle and is one of the most commonly injured nerves during forehead and temporal surgical dissection. The temporal, zygomatic, and buccal divisions all innervate the orbicularis oculi, with significant overlap of regions innervated by each nerve.

REFERENCES

1. Westmore, MG. *Facial cosmetics in conjunction with surgery*, in *Aesthetic Plastic Surgical Society Meeting*. 1975. Vancouver, British Columbia.

2. Gunter, JP, Antrobus, SP, *Aesthetic analysis of the eyebrows*. Plast Reconstr Surg, 1997. **99**: p. 1808–1816.

3. Bosniak, SL, Zilkha, MC, *Cosmetic blepharoplasty and facial rejuvenation*. 1999, Philadelphia: Lippincott-Raven.

4. Lemke, BN, Stasior, OG, *The anatomy of eyebrow ptosis*. Arch Ophthalmol, 1982. **100**: p. 981–986.

5. Tarbet, KJ, Lemke, BN, *Clinical anatomy of the upper face*. Ophthalmol Clin, 1997. **37**: p. 11–28.

6. Kikkawa, DL, Lemke, BN, *Orbital and eyelid anatomy*, in *Ophthalmic Plastic Surgery: Prevention and Management of Complications*, Dortzbach, RK, Editor. 1994, Raven Press: New York.

7. Stasior, GO, Lemke, BN, Wallow, IH, Dortzbach, RK, *Levator aponeurosis elastic fiber network*. Ophthalmic Plast Reconstr Surg, 1993. **9**: p. 1–10.

8. Gavaris, P, *The lid crease [Editor's note]*. Adv Ophthalmic Plast Reconstr Surg, 1982. **1**: p. 89–93.

9. Meyer, D, Linberg, JV, Wobig, JL, McCormick, SA, *Anatomy of the orbital septum and associated eyelid connective tissues: implications for ptosis surgery*. Ophthalmic Plast Reconstr Surg, 1991. **7**: p. 104–113.

10. Jeong, S, Lemke, BN, Dortzbach, RK, Park, YG, Kang, KH, *The Asian upper eyelid: an anatomical study with comparison to the Caucasian eyelid*. Arch Ophthalmol, 1999. **117**: p. 901–912.

11. Doxanas, MT, Anderson, RL, *Oriental eyelids: an anatomic study*. Arch Ophthalmol, 1984. **102**: p. 1232–1235.

12. Hawes, MJ, Dortzbach, RK, *The microscopic anatomy of the lower eyelid retractors*. Arch Ophthalmol, 1982. **100**: p. 1313–1318.

13. Wulc, AE, Dryden, RM, Khatchaturian, T, *Where is the grey line?* Arch Ophthalmol, 1987. **105**: p. 1092–1098.

14. Anderson, RL, Dixon, RS, *The role of Whitnall's ligament in ptosis surgery*. Arch Ophthalmol, 1979. **97**: p. 705.

15. Wesley, RE, McCord, CD, Jones, NA, *Height of the tarsus of the lower eyelid.* Am J Ophthalmol, 1980. **90**: p. 102–105.

16. Scheie, HG, Albert, DM, *Distichiasis and trichiasis: origin and management.* Am J Ophthalmol, 1966. **61**: p. 718–720.

17. Lemke, BN, Della Roca, RC, *Surgery of the eyelids and orbit: an anatomical approach.* 1990, East Norwalk, CT: Appleton & Lange.

18. Dutton, J, *Atlas of clinical and surgical orbital anatomy.* 1994, Philadelphia: WB Saunders Company.

19. Anderson, RL, *The medial canthal tendon branches out.* Arch Ophthalmol, 1977. **95**: p. 2051–2052.

20. Whitnall, SE, *Anatomy of the human orbit.* 1932, London: Oxford University Press.

21. van den Bosch, WA, Leenders, I, Mulder, P, *Topographic anatomy of the eyelids, and the effects of sex and age.* Br J Ophthalmol, 1999. **83**: p. 347–352.

22. Goldberg, RA, Wu, JC, Jesmanowicz, A, Hyde, JS, *Eyelid anatomy revisited: dynamic high-resolution images of Whitnall's ligament and upper eyelid structures with the use of a surface coil.* Arch Ophthalmol, 1992. **110**: p. 1598.

23. Codere, F, Tucker, NA, Renaldi, B, *The anatomy of Whitnall ligament.* Ophthalmology, 1995. **102**: p. 2011–2019.

24. Jones, LT, *An anatomical approach to the problems of the eyelids and lacrimal apparatus.* Arch Ophthalmol, 1961. **105**: p. 1092–1098.

25. Doane, M, *Blinking and the mechanics of the lacrimal drainage system.* Ophthalmology, 1981. **88**: p. 844–851.

26. Jones, LT, *Epiphora: its causes and new surgical procedures for its course.* Am J Ophthalmol, 1954. **38**: p. 824–831.

27. Hill, JC, *Treatment of epiphora owing to flaccid eyelids.* Arch Ophthalmol, 1979. **97**: p. 323–324.

28. Dortzbach, RK, Sutula, FC, *Involutional blepharoptosis: a histopathological study.* Arch Ophthalmol, 1980. **98**: p. 2045–2049.

29. Jones, LT, Quickert, MH, Wobig, JL, *The cure of ptosis by aponeurotic repair.* Arch Ophthalmol, 1975. **93**: p. 629–634.

30. Morton, AD, Elner, VM, Lemke, BN, White, VA, *Lateral extensions of the Müller muscle.* Arch Ophthalmol, 1996. **100**: p. 1486–1488.

31. Bang, YH, Park, SH, Kim, JH, Cho, JH, Lee, CJ, Roh, TS, *The role of Müller's muscle reconsidered.* Plast Reconstr Surg, 1998. **101**: p. 1200–1204.

32. Sires, BS, Lemke, BN, Dortzbach, RK, Gonnering, RS, *Characterization of human orbital fat and connective tissue.* Ophthalmic Plast Reconstr Surg, 1998. **14**: p. 403–414.

33. Knize, DM, *A study of the supraorbital nerve.* Plast Reconstr Surg, 1995. **96**: p. 564–569.

2

ENTROPION

Entropion, or inward rotation of the eyelid margin, is an eyelid malposition commonly seen by general ophthalmologists and oculoplastic surgeons. The severe corneal irritation secondary to contact with the lashes and keratinized epithelium of the eyelid skin brings patients in for evaluation promptly. There are four major types of entropion: congenital, acute spastic, involutional, and cicatricial. It is important to define the pathologic process in entropion to plan and achieve successful surgical repair.

EXAMINATION

A patient with any type of entropion will have complaints related to corneal irritation. Foreign body sensation, redness, and tearing are common. Entropion as well as its symptoms may be intermittent. A careful examination of the lids, lashes, conjunctiva, and cornea should exclude external disease that may exacerbate or cause spastic entropion.

The eyelid examination is first performed like an ectropion exam, in which the canthal tendons, lower lid laxity measurements, and snapback are assessed. In addition, the movement of the lower lid with downgaze may show evidence of weakness of the lower lid retractors. Normal excursion of the lower lid on downgaze is about 4 mm. The depth of the inferior cul-de-sac is assessed and inspected for scarring or symblepharon formation. If there is a cicatricial component to the entropion, this posterior lamellar shortening should be evident with examination. It is important to document the presence or absence of symblepharon, and to diagnose and treat ocular cicatricial pemphigoid prior to surgical intervention. A deep inferior cul-de-sac, or a visible white line (lower lid retractors) several millimeters inferior to the lower tarsal border is consistent with an involutional process.

CONGENITAL ENTROPION-EPIBLEPHARON

Etiology

True congenital entropion is a rare condition in which the entire lid margin is turned in. This is thought to be due to an overacting orbicularis muscle with congenital disinsertion of the lower eyelid retractors. Epiblepharon is much more commonly seen. This condition results from a fold of lower eyelid skin pushing the lashes in against the globe. Epiblepharon is most common in Asian children, and it often resolves as the facial bones develop.

Surgical Management

Congenital entropion can be repaired by reattachment of the capsulopalpebral fascia. This procedure is described in the involutional entropion section, and is performed without concomitant horizontal lid tightening in children.

Epiblepharon repair is necessary if there is evidence of keratopathy or if it is symptomatic. This can be accomplished without any skin removal, in most cases. A horizontal incision is made 1.5 mm below the lash line, across the lower eyelid. The incision should extend a mininum of 2 mm medial and lateral to the inturned area. A small amount of pretarsal orbicularis muscle is removed, to expose the inferior tarsal border. The wound is then closed by approximating the upper skin edge to the inferior tarsal border, and then to the lower skin edge using interrupted 6-0 plain gut suture (Figure 2-1).

ACUTE SPASTIC ENTROPION

Etiology

Spastic entropion, an acute condition that often occurs following eye surgery, injury, or inflammation, is believed to be the direct re-

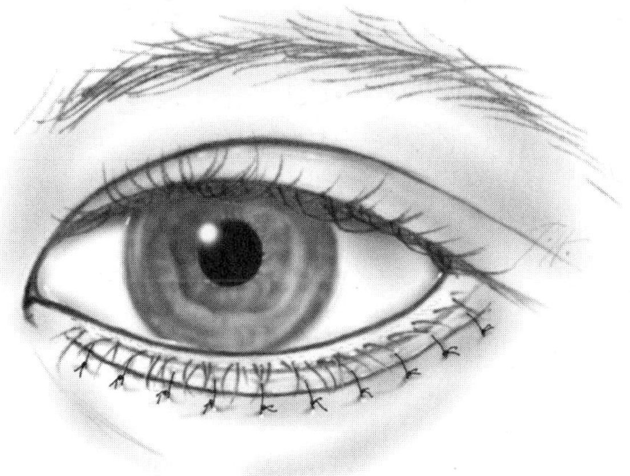

sult of edema and blepharospasm. The process may improve or resolve with resolution of the underlying irritative process, but it may also cause a vicious cycle in which the spastic entropion creates more irritation and more orbicularis spasm. Injection of botulinum toxin is often effective in paralyzing the orbicularis and breaking the cycle. The effect of the botulinum toxin lasts only about 3 months, but the entropion may not recur when the effect wears off. More often than not, the authors have found, there is an underlying involutional component to the spastic entropion and these patients will develop involutional entropion later.

INVOLUTIONAL ENTROPION

Etiology

The most common type of entropion is the involutional type. The pathophysiology of this disorder involves several different mechanisms. Laxity of the medial and lateral canthal tendons, and thinning of the tarsus with aging, result in loss of horizontal support of the lower eyelid. Though a similar process occurs with involutional ectropion, associated dehiscence or attenuation of the lower eyelid retractors creates an imbalance of forces on the tarsus that results in an entropion. Additional contributing factors are thought to include the propensity of the preseptal orbicularis to override the pretarsal orbicularis. Involutional enophthalmos secondary to fat atrophy may contribute, as well, but this has not been proven.

Surgical Management

Capsulopalpebral Fascia Reattachment

The method of repair of entropion is based on the type and severity of the problem, as well as the patient's ability to tolerate a procedure. Involutional entropion is reliably treated with a procedure that addresses the causative factors of the process. After local anesthesia, a subciliary incision is made 2 mm below the lash line from below the punctum to the lateral canthal angle (Figure 2-2). A small skin flap is dissected inferiorly over the tarsus, and a strip of pretarsal orbicularis muscle is dissected off the tarsus. The orbital septum is tented and incised, exposing the thin white edge of capsulopalpebral fascia. This lies below the inferior orbital fat pads, as it is the lower eyelid analogue to the levator. It is useful to mark the fascia with a 4-0 silk suture. A lateral tarsal strip operation is then performed to address the lower eyelid laxity (see Chapter 3) and the strip is sutured to the lateral orbital rim, with the appropriate amount of tension on the eyelid (Figure 2-3). Three or more 6-0 silk sutures are used to reattach the capsulopalpebral fascia (CPF) to the inferior tarsal border (Figure 2-4). The eyelid should not be overcorrected, and the amount of CPF advancement can be confirmed by having the patient look down. The lid should have a normal 3–4 mm excursion. The skin is closed with interrupted 6-0 plain gut suture, and a small amount of CPF edge should be incorporated into the three central sutures to form a barrier to prevent overriding of the orbicularis muscle. The lateral canthal angle is reformed with 6-0 plain gut suture.

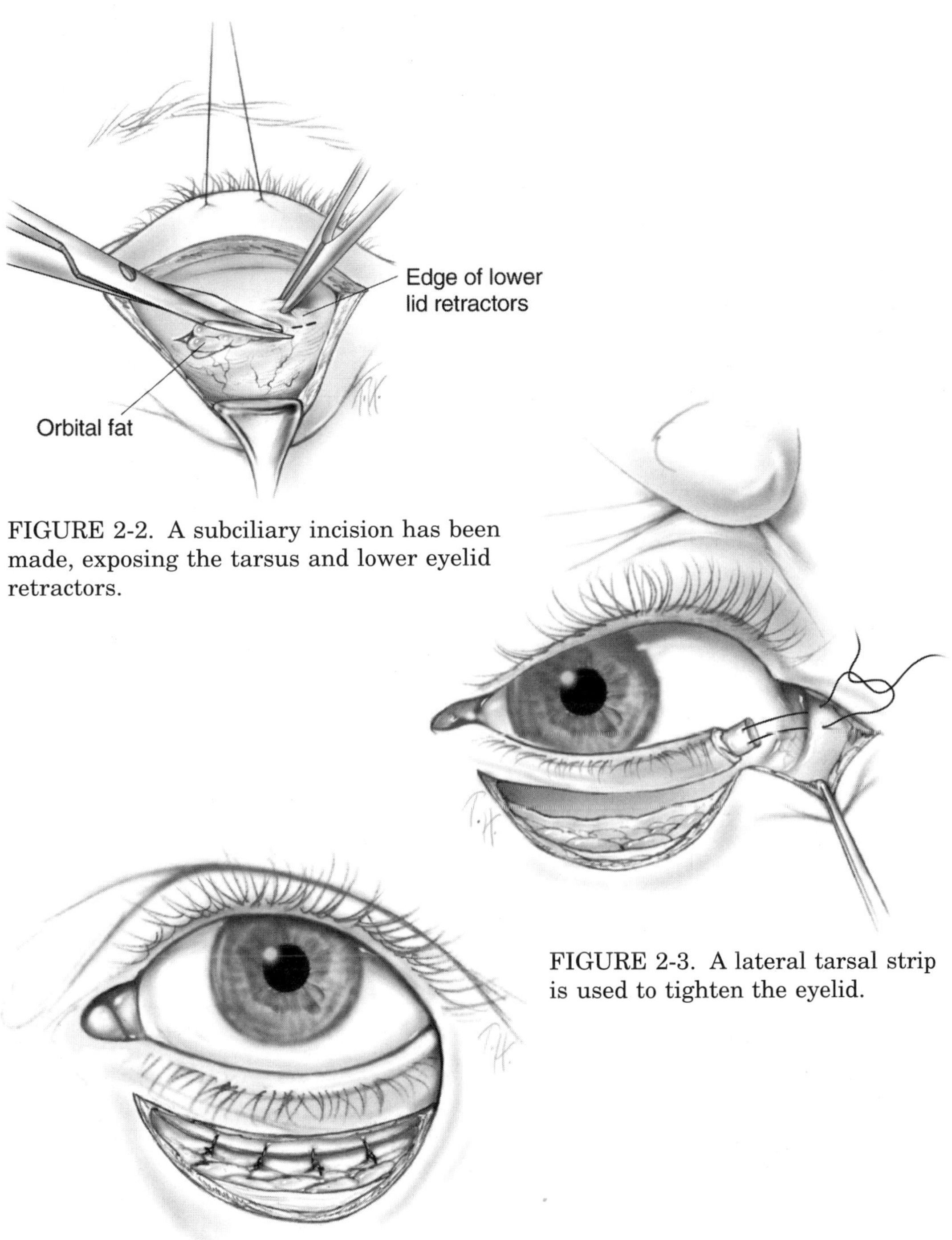

FIGURE 2-2. A subciliary incision has been made, exposing the tarsus and lower eyelid retractors.

FIGURE 2-3. A lateral tarsal strip is used to tighten the eyelid.

FIGURE 2-4. The capsulopalpebral fascia is reattached to the inferior tarsal border.

Quickert Sutures

If a patient who has involutional entropion is a poor surgical candidate, a Quickert, or three-suture, technique can provide relief. However, the recurrence rate is high. Three double-armed 5-0 chromic gut sutures are placed in horizontal mattress fashion 3 mm wide in the lateral, central, and medial lower eyelid. The sutures are passed from deep within the fornix to just beneath the inferior tarsal border as they exit the skin (Figures 2.5 and 2.6). Each suture is tightened to a slight overcorrection.

CICATRICIAL ENTROPION

Etiology

Cicatricial entropion results from a differential horizontal shortening of the posterior lamella of the eyelid in relation to the anterior lamella. Chronic inflammation such as meibomianitis or blepharoconjunctivitis can lead to lid margin keratinization, trichiasis, or distichiasis with severe symptoms in the absence of frank entropion. Trauma, particularly chemical burns, can lead to severe scarring and entropion. Chronic use of medication such as pilocarpine can cause conjunctival contracture leading to entropion. Trachoma is a common cause of entropion internationally, though it is seldom seen in North America. Other causes include ocular cicatricial pemphigoid, severe viral conjunctivitis, and erythema multiforme major (Stevens-Johnson syndrome).

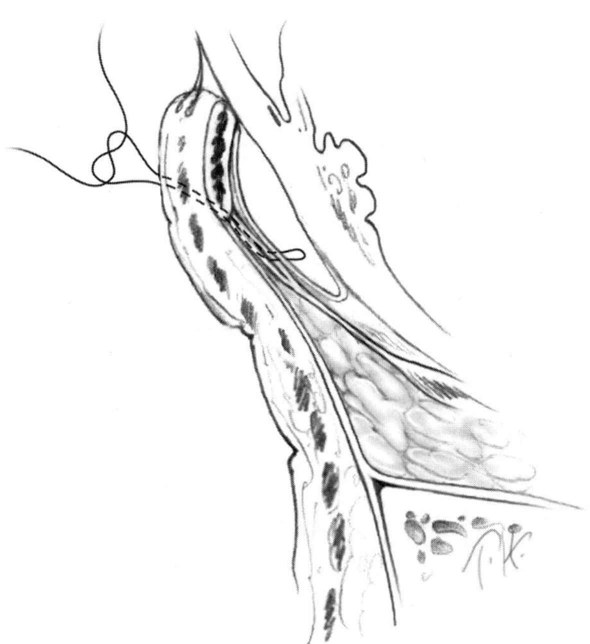

FIGURE 2-5. The suture is passed from the cul-de-sac outward and superiorly.

FIGURE 2-6. When the sutures are tied, the eyelid rotates externally.

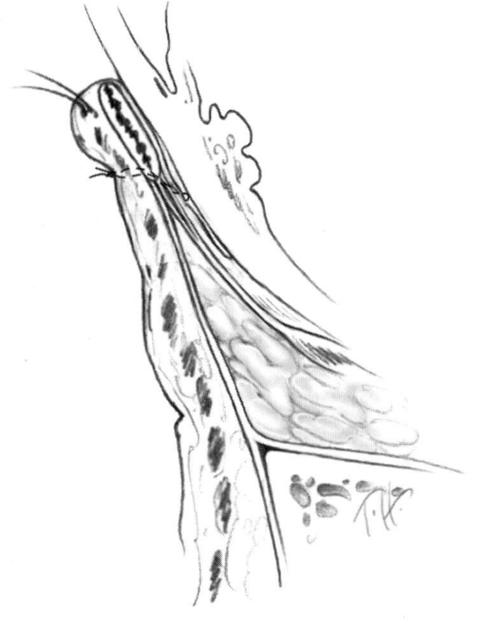

Surgical Management: Wies Procedure

If the entropion is cicatricial in origin, a transverse blepharotomy and marginal rotation (Wies procedure) is effective for repair of the upper or lower eyelid. Local anesthesia is administered to the eyelid, and a horizontal incision is made 4 mm from the lid through skin and orbicularis. Care is taken to spare the marginal arcade, which lies 2–4 mm from the eyelid margin. (Figure 2-7). The lid is then everted, and a second corresponding incision is made through conjunctiva and tarsus. Westcott or tenotomy scissors are used to extend the full-thickness blepharotomy medially and laterally across the tarsus. Three double-armed 6-0 silk sutures are passed in mattress fashion through the tarsus internally, and over the surface of the tarsus to exit the skin near the lash line (Figures 2-8 and 2-9). The closer these sutures are passed to the lashes, the more rotation is achieved. The sutures are tied over cotton or rubber bolsters to prevent "cheese

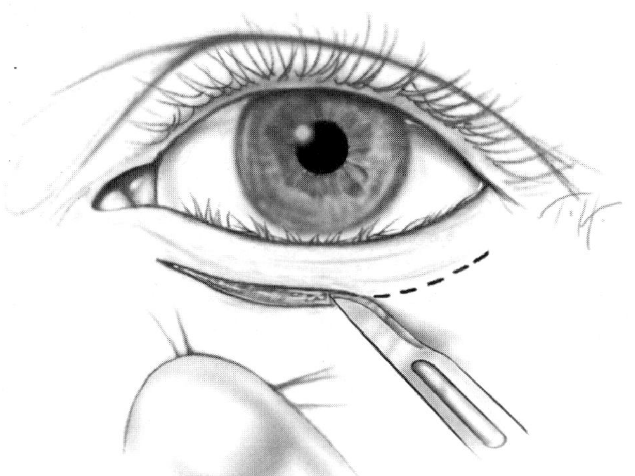

FIGURE 2-7. A skin incision is made
4 mm below the eyelid margin.

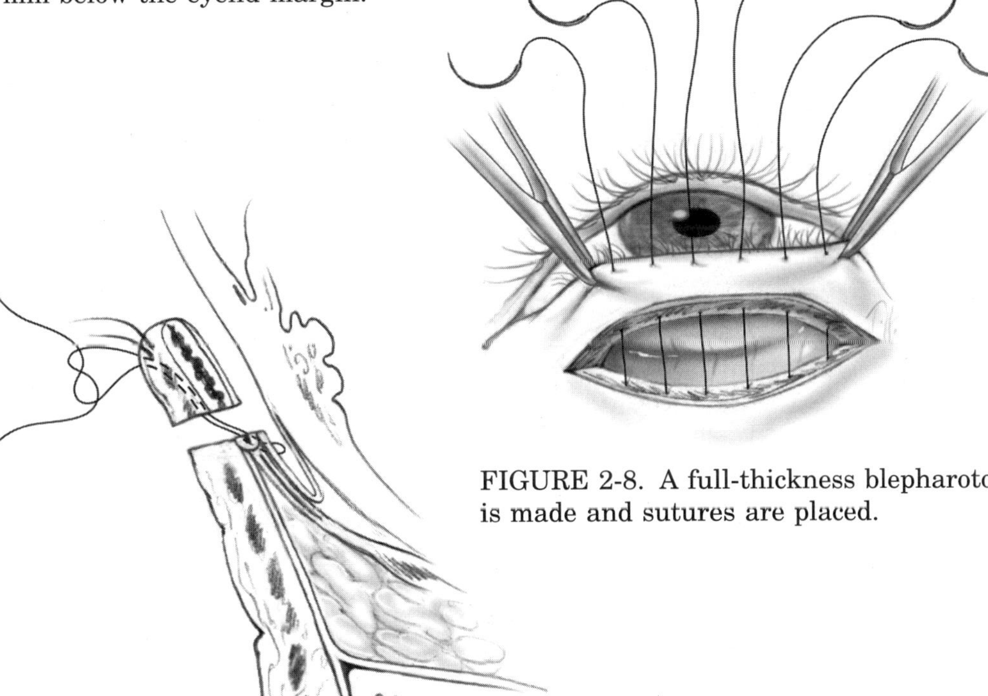

FIGURE 2-8. A full-thickness blepharotomy
is made and sutures are placed.

FIGURE 2-9. Sutures for a full-thickness
blepharotomy.

wiring" (Figure 2-10). A small overcorrection is the goal. The skin incision is closed with interrupted 6-0 plain gut suture. The sutures and bolsters should be removed in 10–14 days.

If the cicatricial entropion is severe, or if the foregoing procedure fails, posterior lamellar augmentation is necessary. A graft may be placed between the conjunctiva/lower lid retractor complex and the inferior tarsal border of the lower lid. The various graft materials available include ear cartilage, hard palate, nasal septum, and mucous membrane grafts. Upon release of the scarring, and production of a posterior lamellar defect, the graft material is sutured into place with absorbable suture and the lid is allowed to heal with a traction suture placing it on stretch. The disadvantage of posterior lamellar grafting is that the lid may not retract well with downgaze.

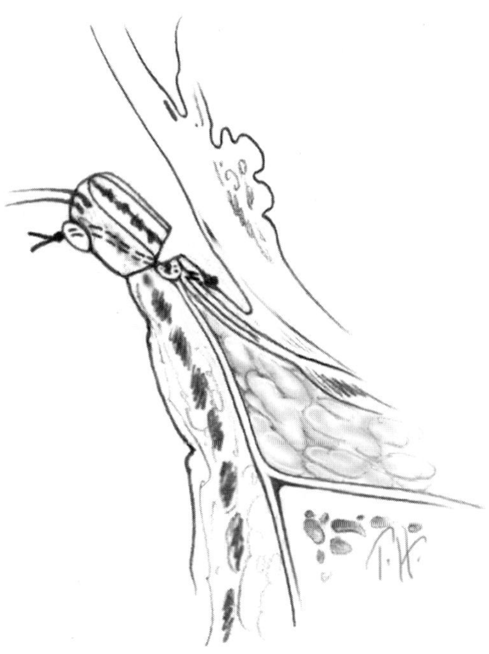

FIGURE 2-10. When the sutures are tied, an external rotation of the eyelid is seen.

3

ECTROPION

Ectropion, or turning out of the eyelid margin, is a common eyelid malposition. Ectropion of the lower eyelid may result from several entirely different pathologic processes. The major types of ectropion are involutional, cicatricial, paralytic, and mechanical. These are all managed differently and are discussed as separate entities.

INVOLUTIONAL ECTROPION

Etiology

As the patient ages, the lower eyelid becomes lax owing to the combination of muscle and tendon atrophy, and gravity. The medial and lateral canthal tendons stretch, and the orbicularis muscle weakens. This creates an imbalance of forces on the tarsal plate, and the eyelid loses its ability to approximate the contour of the globe. The exposed conjunctiva and cornea can become irritated and inflamed. The loss of muscle tone and the eyelid malposition also may result in tearing. The entire process is progressive, and it may be exacerbated by eye rubbing. If the ectropion is long-standing, there may also be a cicatricial component that has developed as a result of shortening of the anterior lamella of the eyelid.

Evaluation

The relationship of the individual anatomic changes must be evaluated to devise a successful treatment plan for ectropion. Most of the data can be obtained by performing the three P's: pinching, pulling, and pushing. The lower eyelid skin is gently pinched, and the eyelid is distracted straight out away from the globe. The distance between the lid and the globe is measured and documented as "lower eyelid laxity." Six millimeters or less is considered normal. The lid is then pulled medially and laterally to evaluated the laxity of the canthal tendons. As the lateral canthal tendon is stretched, the horizontal palpebral width will decrease if the tendon is lax. With tension on the medial canthal tendon, punctal displacement across the nasal limbus will occur when significant laxity is present. Finally, the lid is pushed superiorly. The eyelid margin should easily cross 2–3 mm above the inferior limbus with the eyes in primary gaze. Inferior scleral show and distance of corneal light reflex to lower eyelid margin (MRD$_2$) should be measured as well.

Surgical Management

Lateral Canthal Tendon Plication

The surgical treatment for involutional ectropion depends on the severity of the dysfunction as well as the presence or absence of medial canthal tendon laxity. For mild involutional ectropion without significant medial canthal tendon laxity, a plication of the lateral canthal tendon is effective. This is a minimally invasive procedure that avoids disrupting the canthal angle. After administration of local anesthetic, a subciliary incision is made at the extreme lateral portion of the lower lid and slightly curved to extend out 8–10 mm directly lateral to the lateral canthus (Figure 3-1). The periosteum of the lateral orbital rim is exposed by deeper dissection with scissors or cautery. The inferior crus of the lateral canthal tendon is identified and a double-armed 5-0 Prolene suture is placed through it in a mattress fashion. Each arm of the suture is then threaded through the periosteum of the the inner aspect of the rim. The suture is tied to a moderate amount of tension, and the surgeon should test the tightness of the lid with a gentle pull. A distraction of 2–4 mm is ideal, as this will loosen with time. To help ensure coverage of the permanent suture, the muscle may be closed with inverted interrupted 6-0 Vicryl suture. The skin is closed with 6-0 plain gut suture.

Lateral Tarsal Strip

For repair of moderate to severe generalized ectropion without medial canthal tendon laxity, a lateral tarsal strip procedure is ideal. Local anesthesia is given. A lateral canthotomy is performed by crushing the canthus with a hemostat and making a 10 mm incision straight out from the canthal angle with Westcott scissors (Figure 3-2). The in-

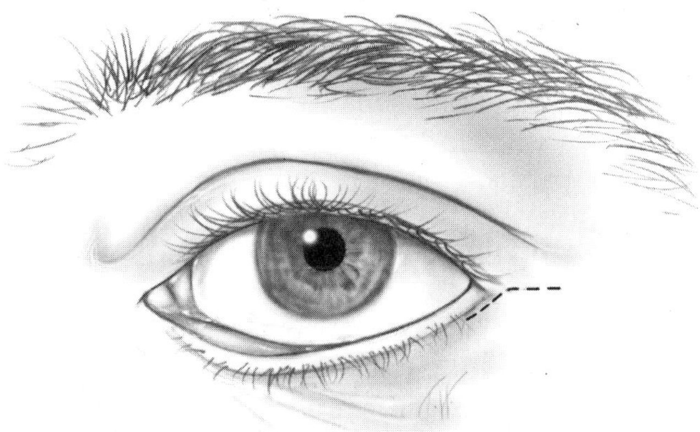

FIGURE 3-1. A lateral canthal skin incision is marked for a lateral canthal tendon plication.

FIGURE 3-2. A lateral canthotomy is made with scissors.

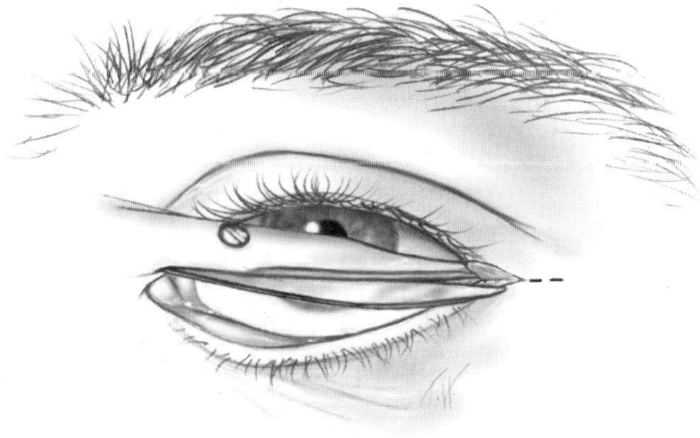

ferior crus of the lateral canthal tendon is identified with palpation
by the tips of the scissors. The tendon is cut, freeing the lateral portion of the lower lid. The length of the strip can then be premarked
by pulling the edge of the lid laterally and marking with a #11 blade
the point on the lid margin where it crosses the interior edge of the
lateral orbital rim. The lid margin and lashes are removed over this
region with the #11 blade (Figure 3-3). A skin muscle flap is dissected
off the anterior tarsal surface of the segment with scissors (Figure
3-4). Along the inferior tarsal border of the segment, scissors are used
to make an incision through conjunctiva and lower lid retractors. The
blade should be used to de-epithelialize the conjunctiva on the posterior surface of the segment. A vertical incision with scissors com-
pletes the creation of the strip by trimming the tarsal strip to a length
of 2–3 mm. Dissection to the periosteum of the lateral orbital rim is
then carried out with scissors and blunt dissection to obtain good vi-

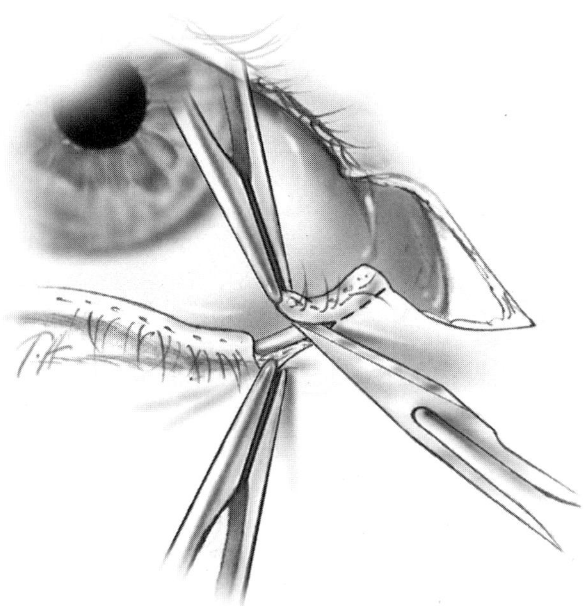

FIGURE 3-3. The eyelid margin is removed, including the lashes.

FIGURE 3-4. Skin and orbicularis are dissected from the anterior tarsal surface.

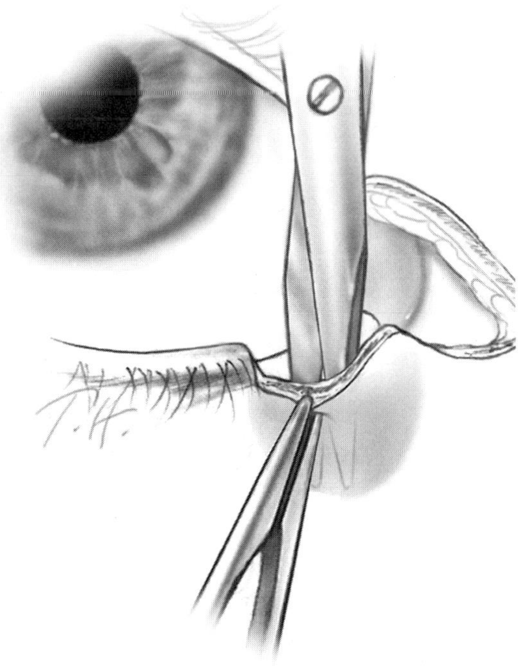

sualization (Figure 3-5). Both arms of a double-armed 5-0 Prolene mattress suture are passed through the tarsal strip, from posterior to anterior, and then through the periosteum (Figure 3-6). In most cases, the periosteal bite should be directed superotemporally. The suture is then tied to an appropriate tension, so the lid can still be distracted 2–4 mm off the globe. The lateral canthal angle is reformed with a single 6-0 plain gut suture, using a circular suture technique to bury the knot in the wound. The muscle and skin are closed with 6-0 Vicryl and 6-0 plain gut, respectively.

Medial Canthal Tendon Plication
If there is significant medial canthal tendon laxity, this condition should be addressed because either of the aforementioned procedures will pull the punctum far laterally. We recommend a minimally invasive, posterior approach to medial canthal tendon plication. This procedure also works well for isolated punctal ectropion with medial canthal tendon laxity. This is accomplished by incising a diamond shape or ellipse of conjunctiva and lower lid retractor tissue 4 mm inferior to the punctum (Figure 3-7). The ellipse should be about 6 mm in length and 3–4 mm in height. Through this ellipse, Westcott scissors are used to bluntly dissect a tunnel to the posterior lacrimal crest. Care is taken to avoid the lacrimal canaliculi and sac. Once the crest has been identified by palpation and dissection, both needles of a double-armed 5-0 Prolene suture are passed through the inferomedial edge of the tarsus that has been exposed through the elliptical incision, from anterior to posterior. A forceps is then passed into the tunnel and the medial canthal tendon attachment to the posterior

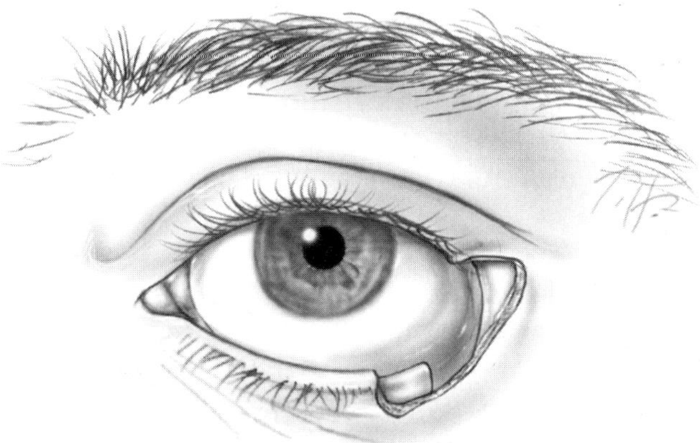

FIGURE 3-5. The lateral orbital rim periosteum
is exposed.

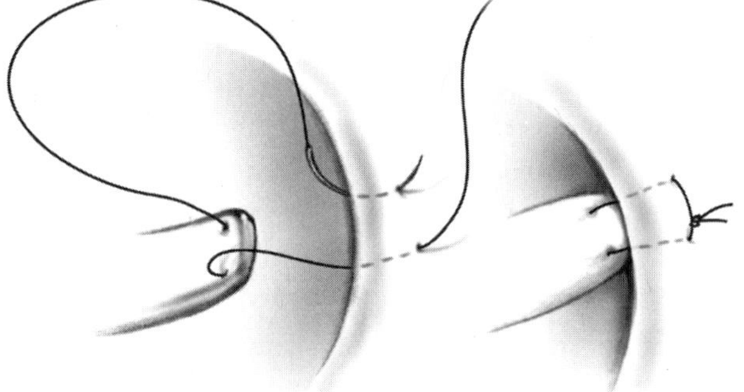

FIGURE 3-6. A mattress suture fas-
tens the tarsal strip to the periosteum.

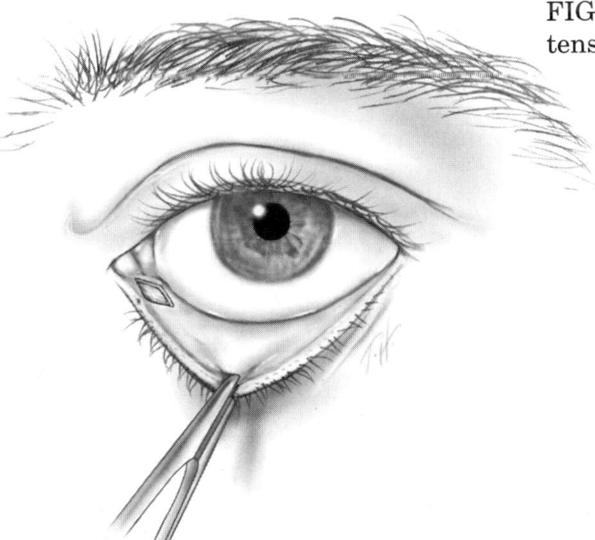

FIGURE 3-7. A diamond-shaped excision of
conjunctiva and retractors is performed.

lacrimal crest is grasped and exposed (Figure 3-8). Each arm of the mattress suture is passed through this tissue, and the suture is tied to the appropriate tension. Closure of the elliptical incision with interrupted, buried 6-0 plain gut suture will further facilitate inward rotation of the punctum to complete the medial ectropion repair.

Medial Ectropion Repair

Punctal ectropion with normal medial canthal tendon function can be repaired with a similar elliptical excision to shorten the posterior lamella. The conjunctiva and lid retractor tissue are excised, as done earlier, and the ellipse is closed by a double-armed 6-0 chromic gut or Vicryl suture. The suture is passed in mattress fashion, from anterior to posterior, through the upper portion of the wound (the inferior tarsal border edge). Each needle is then passed through the lower wound edge, from posterior to anterior. Finally, the needles are passed through the center of the ellipse and out the skin of the lower lid, existing more inferiorly than they entered. They are then tied (Figure 3-9). This rotates the punctum inward, completing the procedure.

Cases of extreme or refractory ectropion may require more extensive surgery, such as combination tarsal strip and pentagonal wedge resection, or temporalis muscle transfer procedures. These operations, which are rarely necessary, are not discussed in this volume.

PARALYTIC ECTROPION

Ectropion of the lower lid may result from paralysis of the orbicularis muscle. This may occur with Bell's palsy, trauma, surgery (including facial or parotid gland procedures), or cerebrovascular accident. If the paralysis is permanent, ectropion becomes very likely. The eyes often become irritated and corneal exposure may be a concern. Tearing is common because of lid malposition and loss of pump function. Conservative measures for treatment include vigorous lubrication and moisture chambers, but these usually are not effective for long-term management. A lateral tarsal strip procedure is an effective repair for paralytic ectropion. In cases of severe corneal exposure, a tarsorrhaphy is sometimes necessary.

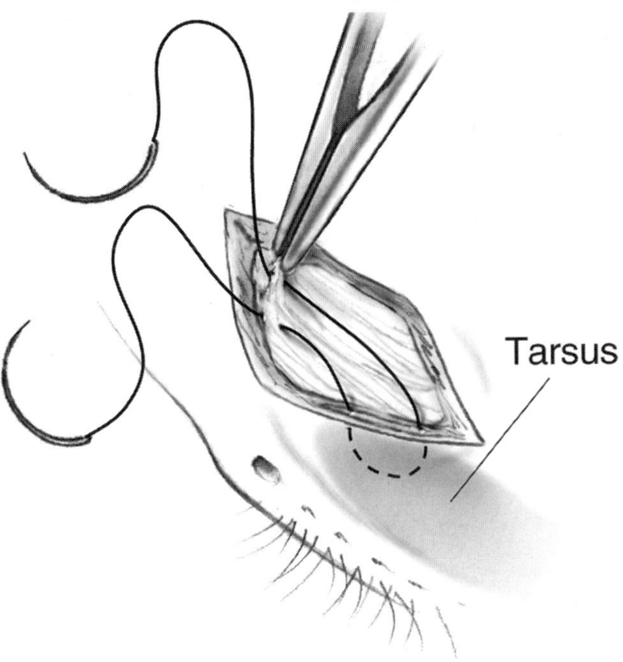

FIGURE 3-8. The medial canthal tendon is plicated with a permanent suture.

FIGURE 3-9. The ellipse is closed, producing an inward rotation of the punctum.

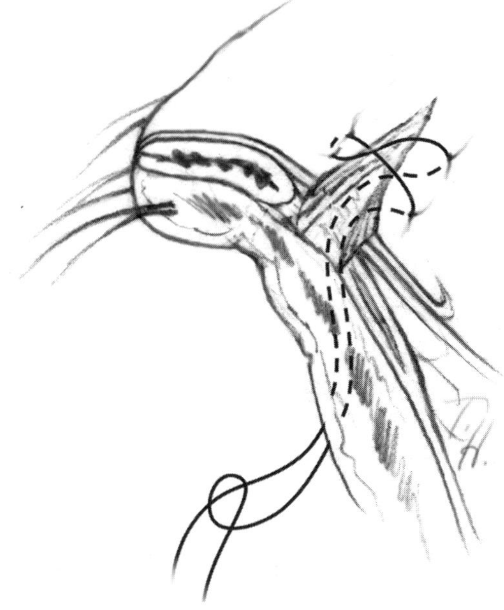

Cicatricial Ectropion

Etiology

Ectropion due to scarring often involves a shortening of the anterior lamella of the eyelid. Scarring from actinic changes or dermatologic conditions may be uniform and can cause a diffuse bilateral ectropion. Trauma can cause random, irregular scarring with segmental or complete ectropion. In any of these cases, the anterior lamellar insufficiency must be addressed for repair to be successful. Full-thickness skin grafting is the main procedure for correcting these abnormalities. Z-plasty has a role in smaller scars and segmental ectropion, but often this procedure does not give the aesthetic result of scar removal with graft.

Surgical Management

The repair of cicatricial ectropion is detailed but technically straightforward. The scar tissue is excised, and any remaining scar bands in the anterior lamella are lysed (Figure 3-10). This is usually facilitated by placing a 4-0 silk traction suture through the lid margin to permit palpation of the bands with the lid on stretch. It is important to free all scarring so that the lid settles in a normal position without tension (Figure 3-11). Once the region containing the scarring is free and mobilized, a defect will remain in the anterior lamella. A piece of Telfa gauze is then blotted over the defect and cut with scissors to the same size. This is the template for the skin graft. A variety of sites can be used to obtain the full-thickness skin graft. For lower eyelid or medial canthal grafts, retroauricular skin gives a good match. Upper eyelid skin, if available, works best for upper lid grafts, but can also be used for lower lids or canthal reconstruction. When upper lid skin is the chosen donor tissue, be sure to verify that adequate skin will remain, and allow eye closure by using a pinch technique. Once the site has been chosen, the donor graft is marked using the Telfa template. A #15 Bard-Parker blade is used to incise the skin, and a thin full-thickness skin graft is removed with Westcott scissors. The graft may be thinned with Westcott scissors to remove excess subcutaneous tissue, and the borders trimmed. Full-thickness eyelid skin grafts shrink only a small amount, if at all, so only slight oversizing is recommended.

The graft is placed in the defect and sutured into place using interrupted 6-0 plain gut suture (Figure 3-12). The ends of four or six of these sutures may be left long, or additional silk sutures may be

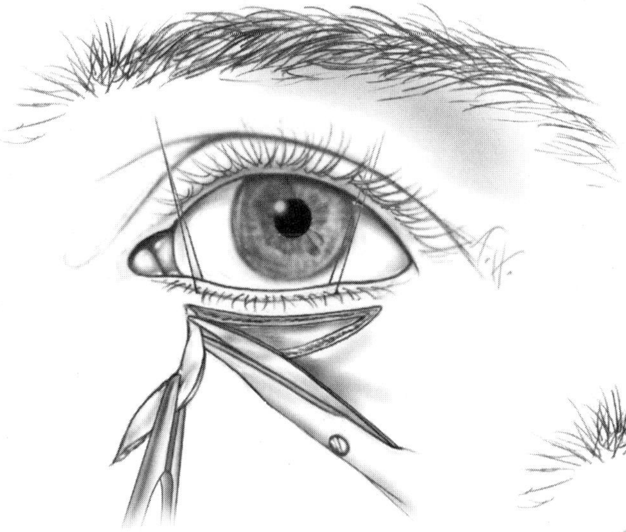

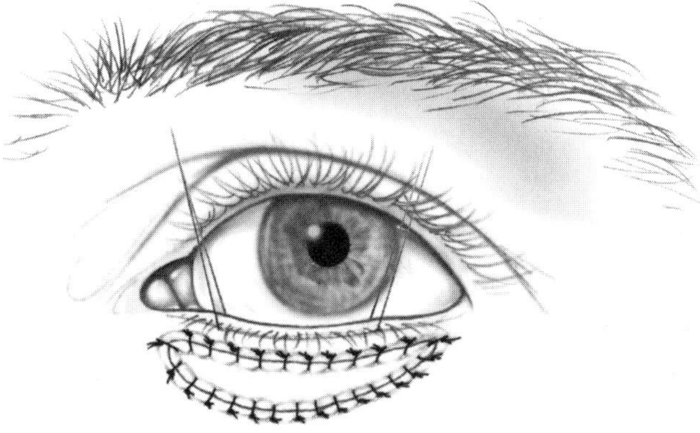

FIGURE 3-10. Superficial scar tissue is excised.

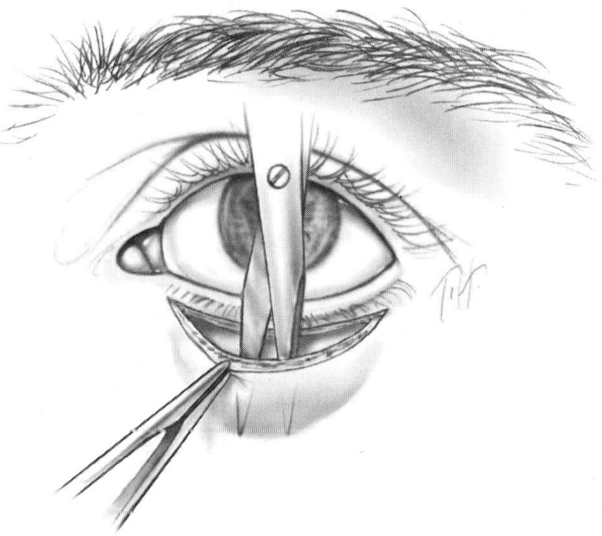

FIGURE 3-11. Scar tissue bands are dissected and removed.

FIGURE 3-12. A skin graft is sutured in place.

placed around the graft to secure a bolster. The Telfa template (or a new one) is placed over the graft and a small, damp piece of cotton is compressed and placed on the Telfa. The sutures are then snugly tied over this bolster to place gentle pressure on the graft against the underlying bed, from which it will receive its blood supply. Unless a large graft (> 4 cm^2) is being placed, fenestration is usually not necessary with this technique. The 4-0 silk traction suture is taped with Mastisol adhesive and Steri-Strip bandages to the forehead (for lower lid traction) or cheek (for upper lid traction) to place the lid on mild stretch. The bolster can be removed in one week.

Mechanical Ectropion

Mechanical ectropion is really a secondary ectropion resulting from an eyelid mass. Any large eyelid tumor or inflammatory mass can cause an ectropion. The treatment is removal of the mass. If the process is long-standing, there may be a residual involutional type of ectropion following mass removal. A pentagonal wedge resection of the mass will often treat both problems effectively. In some cases, additional lid tightening is required.

4

EYELID RETRACTION

Eyelid retraction is a common condition encountered in ophthalmology. Its diagnosis and appropriate management involve a systematic approach beginning with a complete history. It is important for the surgeon to be aware of conditions that could potentially worsen the retraction. A thorough history and physical examination will help the physician avoid misdiagnosis and inappropriate surgical intervention.

ETIOLOGY

There are many conditions responsible for retraction of the eyelid. It is most commonly seen in thyroid-related ophthalmopathy. Cicatricial causes include trauma and surgery. Noncicatricial causes include aberrant regeneration of third nerve, unilateral ptosis with contralateral overaction of levator palpebrae muscle, Collier's sign of dorsal midbrain syndrome (Parinaud's), hyperkalemic periodic paralysis, and chronic systemic corticosteroid therapy.

Aberrant regeneration of the third nerve, or misdirection syndrome, results from injured nerve fibers. As the nerves heal, there may be extensive and haphazard growth. This will result in upper lid retraction on attempted downgaze (Von Graefe's sign). Patients who have unilateral ptosis can present with contralateral upper lid retraction from overaction of the levator palpebrae muscle due to excessive attempt to elevate the ptotic eye. Correction of the ptosis usually will improve the retraction. Dorsal midbrain syndrome, or Parinaud's syndrome, produces a constellation of neuro-ophthalmic signs as a result of lesions in the rostral midbrain. Most common causes are pineal area tumors and midbrain infarction. This can result in a pathological lid retraction (Collier's sign) and lid lag (inability to fully close the eyelid).

Prevalence/Incidence

In patients with Graves disease it is believed that circulating T cells are directed against the cross-reactive antigens in the orbit.[1] These activated T cells and macrophages release cytokines, which stimulate the autoimmune response resulting in the disease. At some point during their diagnosis of Graves disease, 90% of patients will get eyelid retraction. Of those diagnosed, 90% have hyperthyroidism, 1% has hypothyroidism, 3% have Hashimoto thyroiditis, and 6% are euthyroid. It is important to have a good medical evaluation with an endocrinologist.

PATHOPHYSIOLOGY OF UPPER AND LOWER EYELID RETRACTION

The many factors that have been associated with upper lid retraction in patients with thyroid ophthalmopathy include overaction of the levator muscle, increased sympathetic tone causing Müller muscle contraction, proptosis of the globe, fibrosis with contracture of the levator aponeurosis, and adhesions of the levator to the orbital septum. It has been postulated that because of the restrictive myopathic nature of the inferior rectus muscle, the superior rectus-levator complex overcompensates and causes the upper lid to retract (Figure 4-1).

Retraction of the lower lid can result from inferior rectus contracture, over-contraction of the inferior tarsal muscle with increased sympathetic tone, proptosis, and prior surgical recession of the inferior rectus muscle. Cicatricial causes such as trauma and surgery must also be considered.

PREOPERATIVE EVALUATION

The upper eyelid normally is positioned 1.5 mm inferior to the 12 o'clock limbus. The distance between the corneal light reflex and the upper lid margin, MRD_1 (margin reflex distance), is the most useful measurement for documentation and monitoring of eyelid retraction.

Eyelid Retraction

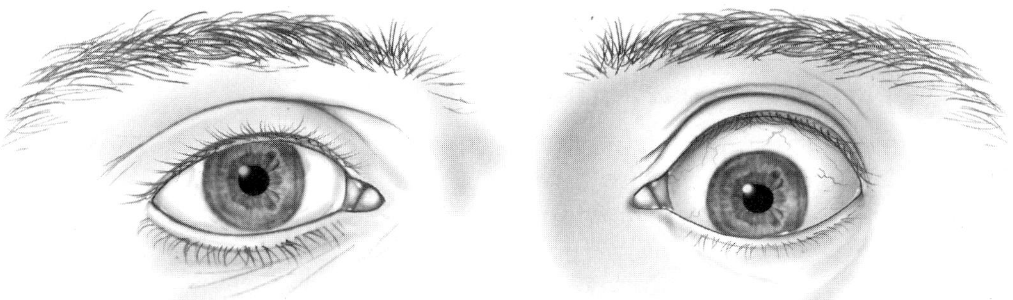

FIGURE 4-1. The left globe is hypotropic, thereby stimulating left upper eyelid retraction, creating a pseudoretraction.

It is sometimes useful to measure MRD_1 with the room lights dim. This will prevent artificially low readings due to photophobia, often present in these patients. A system established by Waller gives a useful grading method for upper lid retraction.[2] Retraction of 1–2 mm is considered mild, 2–5 mm moderate, and greater than 5 mm is severe. The amount of lagophthalmos is documented during gentle lid closure. The cornea is examined closely for signs of exposure keratopathy. A basic secretor test must be performed by installation of proparacaine. At 1 minute the wetting on the filter paper strip should be 5 mm. Preoperative photographs are essential for documentation and for postoperative comparison. It may be useful to obtain a nonenhanced CT scan with axial and direct coronal 3 mm image cuts. This will allow the surgeon to visualize any extraocular muscle enlargement and to rule out other orbital pathology such as vascular or neoplastic entities.

MANAGEMENT: MEDICAL

The most important medical management is with artificial tear lubricants, which can prevent corneal exposure, corneal erosion, and secondary corneal ulcer. Topical sympatholytic agents such as guanethidine, an α-adrenergic blocker, have been introduced in the past.[3] They, however, have not been very useful in managing eyelid retraction. Botulinum A has also been used, but relief is only temporary and ptosis a significant potential side effect.

MANAGEMENT: SURGICAL

Upper Eyelid Retraction

When surgical repair of eyelid retraction is appropriate, the goals are to limit scleral show, minimize lagophthalmos, reduce corneal exposure, and restore a normal appearance. In the upper lid this is achieved by vertically elongating the posterior lamella of the eyelid with levator recession and/or mullerectomy. The decision to proceed with an anterior or posterior approach depends on the surgeon's training and comfort level. The anterior approach provides the surgeon with a familiar anatomical layout, and resuspension of the lacrimal gland can simultaneously be addressed. Also, orbital fat can be debulked through this method. The posterior approach provides less familiar anatomical landmarks and may therefore have a steep learning curve. There is an additional risk of damaging the lacrimal gland ductules through this approach, and bleeding is more common. Because many patients are younger females, the posterior approach has a significant advantage in that it avoids an external incision and eliminates scarring. The patient should be counseled that 2–3 weeks of healing is required before the lid assumes a stable position. Waller states that recession of Müller's muscle can lower the upper eyelid 1.5 mm.[4] Detachment of levator aponeurosis from the anterior aspect of the tarsus will lower the eyelid up to 0.5 mm, and detachment of the subcutaneous insertion of the levator aponeurosis will lower the eyelid 1.5 mm.

Posterior Approach

The patient's MRD_1, lagophthalmos, and palpebral fissure height are measured carefully preoperatively. Surgery via mullerectomy is an outpatient procedure with intravenous sedation and local anesthesia. This surgery should not be done under general anesthesia unless absolutely necessary. Tetracaine eyedrops (0.5–0.1%) are instilled in both eyes. Usually a Diprivan drip is administered. Lidocaine 2% with 1:100,000 epinephrine and 0.5% Marcaine with 1:200,000 epinephrine is given in a 50:50 mixture in a 10 mL syringe on a 27 or 30 gauge needle. Sometimes 1 mL of Wydase (hyaluronic acid) can be added to the mixture to help with diffusion of the anestitetic solution. The upper eyelid is everted and the local anesthetic is administered. To avoid injection to the levator, the anesthetic mixture is injected just beneath the conjunctiva, at the superior tarsal border.

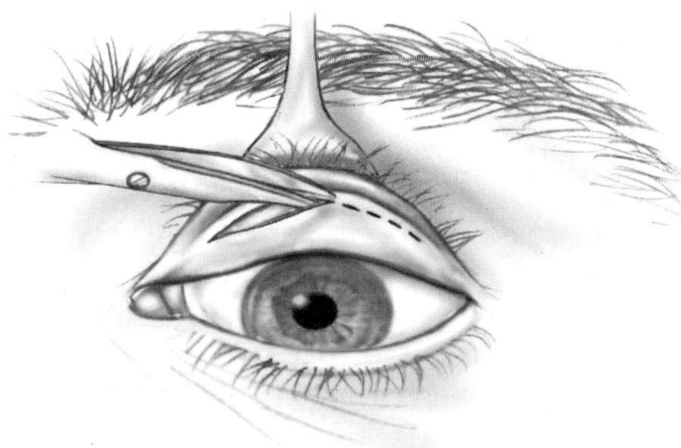

FIGURE 4-2. The conjunctiva is incised at the superior tarsal border over the temporal two-thirds of the eyelid.

This injection also creates a hydrodissection of the conjunctiva from Müller's muscle. A 4-0 silk traction suture is placed through the skin centrally at the lash line of the upper lid. A Desmarres retractor is used to evert the upper eyelid. A buttonhole incision is made temporally through the conjunctiva at the superior border of the tarsus. Westcott scissors are then used to dissect the conjunctiva away from the superior border of the tarsus across the temporal two-thirds of the eyelid (Figure 4-2). In thyroid patients, who have more retraction temporally, the incision usually does not need to extend beyond the medial third of the eyelid. Hemostasis is achieved with pressure, and it is better to avoid too much cauterization to prevent damage to the lacrimal ductules. The conjunctiva is then freed from its attachments to Müller's muscle with Westcott scissors.

Another buttonhole incision is made temporally at the superior border of the tarsus through Müller's muscle. Anatomical awareness of this muscle is fundamental for this surgery. Müller's muscle originates from the undersurface of the levator aponeurosis at Whitnall's ligament, 14–16 mm above the superior border of the tarsus. This sympathetically innervated muscle inserts on the superior border of the tarsus and has some attachments to the conjunctival fornix. Once the buttonhole incision has been made, Müller's muscle is disinserted from the superior tarsal border in the temporal two-thirds of the eyelid. At this point the attachment of Müller's muscle to the levator aponeurosis is carefully separated with blunt and sharp dissection (Figure 4-3). The patient can then sit up to allow the surgeon to determine the height and contour of the upper eyelid. If retraction is still present, the levator aponeurosis is grasped above the superior tarsal border with two forceps gently stretched vertically. Care is taken to avoid damage to the skin (Figure 4-4). This maneuver is titrated by incrementally stretching the levator, and checking lid position until the lid margin is 1 mm below the superior limbus and contour is ideal. Next, the Müller's muscle is infiltrated with the local anesthetic mixture, and a straight hemostat is clamped across the base of the muscle for a few seconds. The muscle is then excised with a high temperature cautery. In some cases, lid height and contour are ideal after initial Müller's detachment. The levator then need not be addressed, and the muscle can be excised. A 6-0 plain gut buried interrupted suture is used to reattach conjunctiva to the superior tarsal border centrally, medially, and laterally. The 4-0 silk is then removed and patient is given ophthalmic ointment with a pressure patch for 24 hours. Postoperative ptosis may be present for about 1 week. The lid should achieve a stable position within 3–4 weeks. There may be a role for downward eyelid massage for persistent retraction in the early postoperative period.

Anterior Approach

The anterior approach for upper eyelid retraction can be performed with or without a lid spacer material placed between the levator aponeurosis and tarsus. Goldstein originally described this approach in 1934.[5] Available spacer materials include auricular cartilage, banked sclera, fascia lata, and most recently AlloDerm.[6] A major advantage of the anterior approach is the familiarity of the anatomy and the preservation of the lacrimal gland ductules. Also, there is less potential irritation of the cornea from conjunctival sutures, which can be a problem with the posterior approach. For the purposes of this chapter and the video, the procedure is described without a lid spacer.

The upper eyelid crease is marked with a marking pen prior to infiltration with 2% lidocaine with epinephrine 1:100,000 and Marcaine with 1:200,000 epinephrine for a 50:50 mixture, in a 10 mL syringe. If desired, 1 mL of Wydase can be added. An incision is made along the marking with a blade. If there is excessive skin, a pinch technique can be used to determine the amount to be excised. Westcott scissors are used to remove skin and part of the preseptal orbicularis. If no skin excision is to be performed, a suborbicularis plane

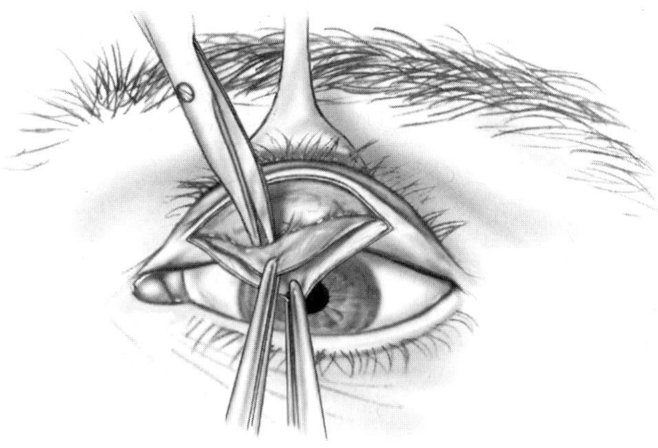

FIGURE 4-3. Müller's muscle is dissected off the levator aponeurosis.

FIGURE 4-4. Two toothed forceps are used to elongate the levator aponeurosis, adjusting both the eyelid height and contour.

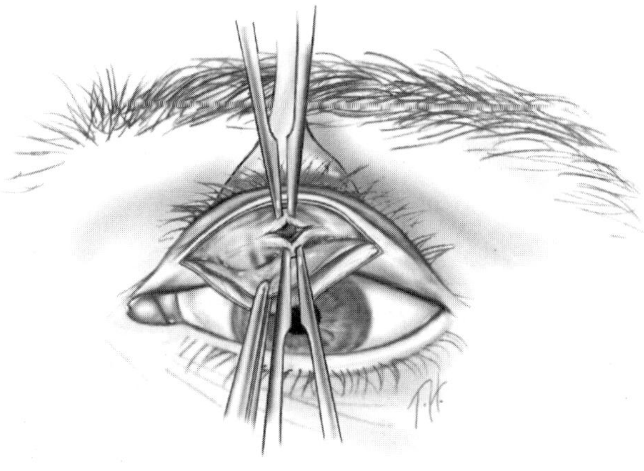

is dissected superior and inferior to the incision. Once the anterior skin muscle flap dissection has been carried inferiorly, a portion of the pretarsal orbicularis is removed, exposing the superior border of the tarsus. While gently pulling the edge of the levator aponeurosis inferiorly and the septum superiorly, the surgeon incises the septum with scissors or cautery. Orbital septum is then opened at a 45° angle cephalad. This plane is important to prevent damage to the levator aponeurosis (Figure 4-5). The lid is everted and the conjunctiva is hydrodissected from the Müller's muscle with 2% lidocaine with epinephrine superior to the tarsal border. The lid is flipped back and the cautery is used to detach Müller's muscle from the superior aspect of the tarsus across the lateral two thirds of the lid (Figure 4-6). Once separated from conjunctiva, the muscle can be either excised or recessed. The temporal horn of the levator aponeurosis can now be recessed until an optimal height is obtained. The patient is asked to open and close the eyes to judge the desired contour and height of the upper lid. We believe the recession of the levator is important to prevent temporal flaring. When the height is satisfactory, the leva-

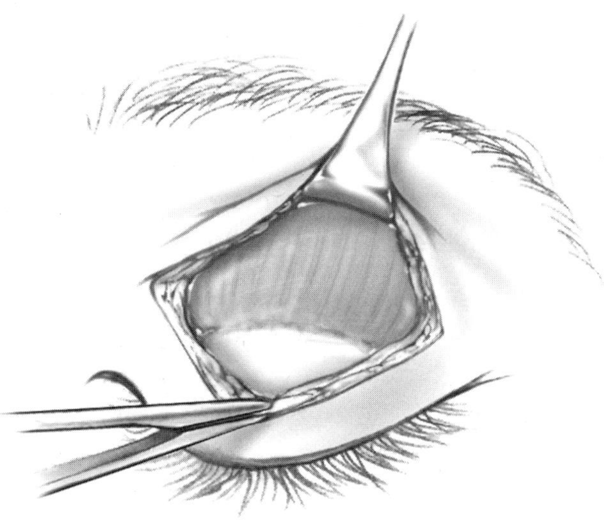

FIGURE 4-5. An external incision is made to identify the levator aponeurosis.

FIGURE 4-6. The levator is detached from the superior border of the tarsus.

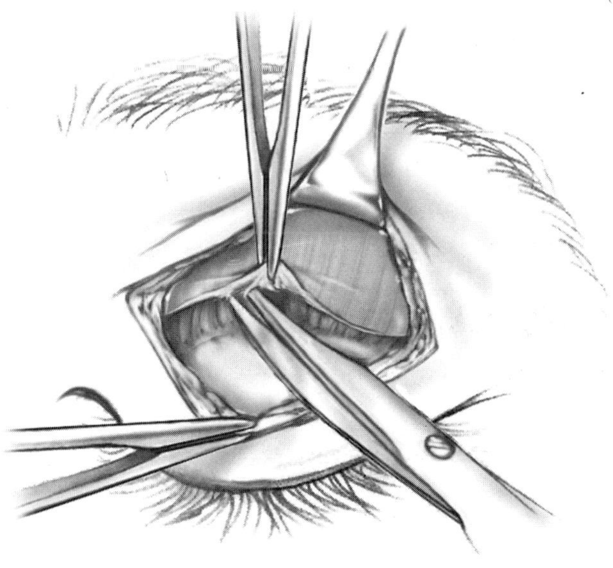

tor is left unsutured. A hangback suture can be placed as well (Figure 4-7). Skin closure is performed with running subcuticular 6-0 Prolene. The sutures are left untied at both ends. Tincture of benzoin and adhesive suture strips are placed along the incision without ointment. The sutures are removed in one week.

When spacer material is used in retraction surgery, it is placed between the levator aponeurosis and the superior border of the tarsus (Figure 4-8). The graft should be wider temporally. Upper eyelid retraction usually does not require spacer grafts, but they are often used for lower lid retraction.

Lower Eyelid Retraction

As in the upper eyelid, lower eyelid retraction can be repaired with either an anterior or posterior approach. We prefer the posterior transconjunctival approach. As stated earlier, donor grafts are usually used. They will give approximately 3–5 mm of elevation on the lower eyelid. The video accompanying this chapter illustrates the use of ear cartilage as the lid spacer graft. Independent of the type of spacer used, the approach is the same. The material is placed between the inferior border of the tarsus and conjunctiva of the inferior fornix. If sclera is used, it is sized to a ratio of 1.5–2.5 mm for each millimeter of elavation. Auricular cartilage and the other materials use a ratio of 1:1. The type of material used depends on availability and the comfort level of the surgeon.

The lower lid, retroauricular area, and preauricular area are infiltrated with 2% Xylocaine with epinephrine 1:100,000, 0.5% Marcaine with 1:200,000 epinephrine, and Wydase if desired for a 50:50 mixture. To harvest the ear cartilage graft, a 4-0 silk traction suture is placed posterior through the skin of the helix to hold the ear forward. The amount of retraction, determined preoperatively, is used to arrive at the width of the ear cartilage. The length of the cartilage is usually 22–25 mm. A straight metal ruler is used to mark 22–25 mm linear area at the flattened portion of the posterior aspect of the

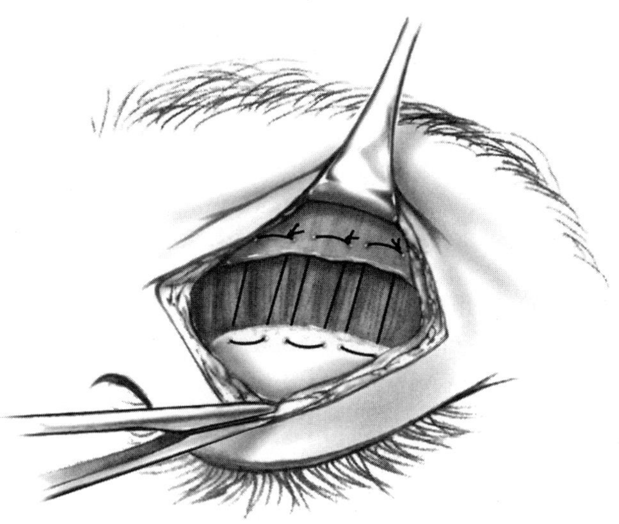

FIGURE 4-7. The levator is recessed with or without a mullerectomy. One to three hangback sutures can be placed.

FIGURE 4-8. An example of upper eyelid lengthening by means of a spacer graft between the superior border of the tarsus and the leading edge of the levator aponeurosis.

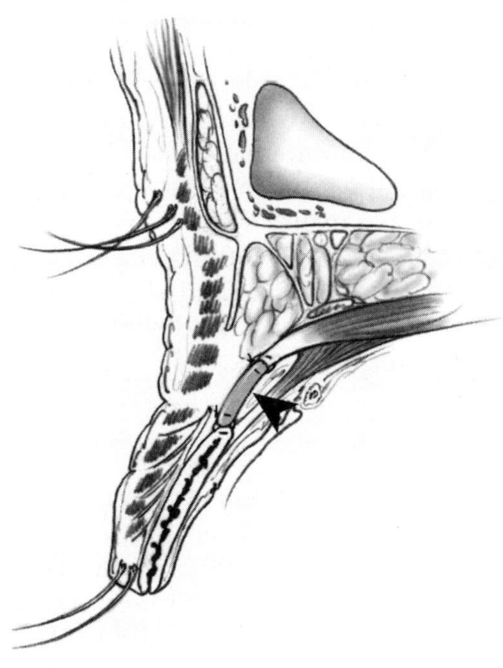

helix at the junction between the ear and the skull (Figure 4-9). An incision is made along the marking. Dissection is carried down to the top of the auricular cartilage. A line 22–25 mm long is marked along the cartilage with cautery. The 1:1 ratio is used to determine the width of the cartilage graft and is marked above and below the straight line in either direction. For example, if the desired width is 4 mm, 2 mm is marked anterior and 2 mm posterior from the center of the cartilage. High temperature cautery is then used to delineate an ellipse of ear cartilage to be excised. A partial-thickness incision is made through the cartilage, and care is necessary to avoid incising the underlying skin. Westcott scissors are then used to excise the graft. The skin of the ear is closed with a running 6-0 plain gut. The cartilage should not be sutured.

Two 4-0 silk traction sutures are placed below the lash line in the lower eyelid. A lateral canthotomy followed by an inferior cantholysis is performed for adequate exposure. The inferior retractor muscles and conjunctiva are disinserted from the inferior border of the tarsus along the length of the lower lid. A dissection is then carried out just anterior to the conjunctiva and retractor muscles (Figure 4-10). When the capsulopalpebral fascia and retractor muscles have been removed from the inferior border of the tarsus, the lid will elevate. The cartilage graft is then placed with the smooth side toward the conjuntiva and sutured with 6-0 chromic gut inferiorly to the conjunctiva and superiorly to the inferior border of the tarsus in interrupted fashion (Figure 4-11). The superior sutures should be inverted to avoid irritation or abrasion. The conjunctiva is then scraped from the lateral tarsal surface. The lateral tarsus is then fixed to the periosteum of the lateral orbital rim with a double-armed 5-0 Prolene suture and tightened to the appropriate lid tension. The tension of the eyelid must not be too tight. The lateral canthal angle is re-formed with a circular suture, and the skin is closed with 6-0 plain gut. The lower lid is pulled up for traction with the 4-0 silk, and this suture is taped above the brow with Steri-Strips to place the lower lid on gentle stretch. This dressing is removed in one week.

CONCLUSION

Surgical repair of eyelid retraction requires careful patient evaluation. Both the timing of the surgery and the type of procedure selected are very important and should be discussed with the patient in detail. It is important to discuss the variability of the eyelid in thy-

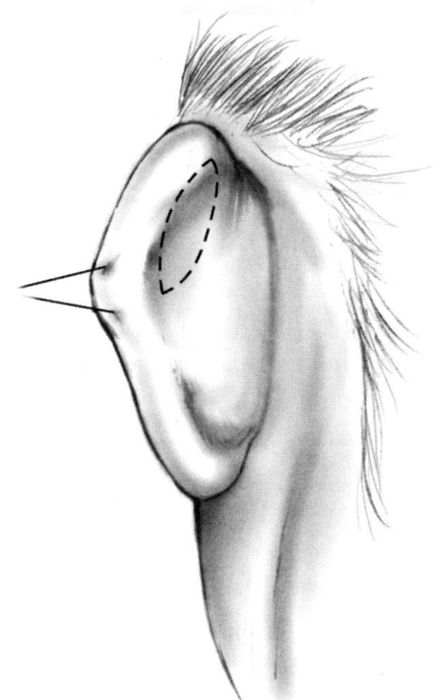

FIGURE 4-9. The flattened portion of the posterior ear just anterior to the helix is used as a donor site for ear cartilage. Dashed lines show a typical ear cartilage graft.

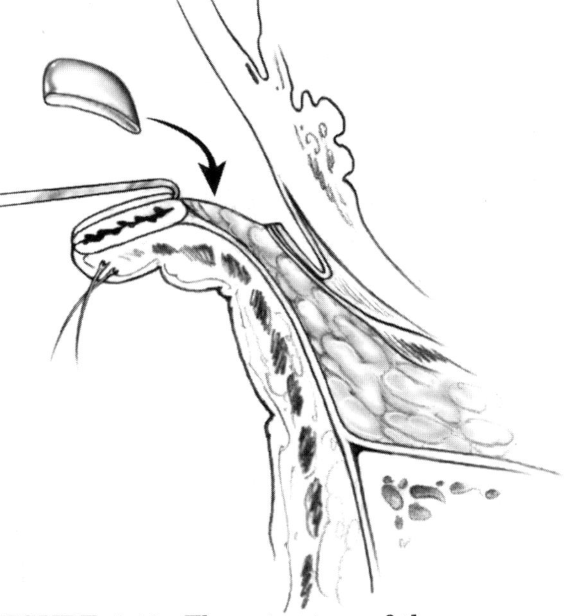

FIGURE 4-10. The retractors of the lower eyelid have been recessed from the inferior tarsal border.

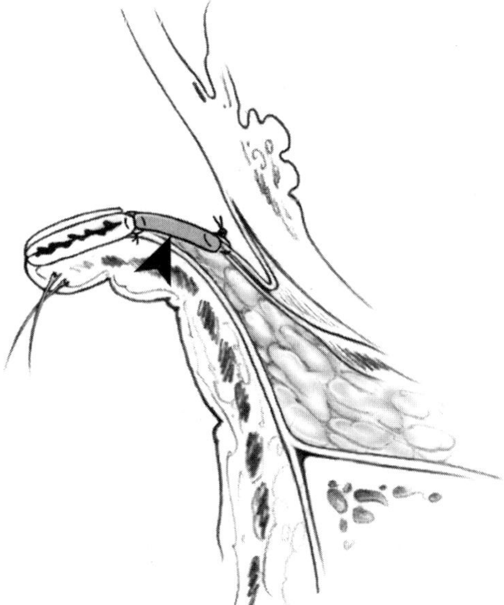

FIGURE 4-11. A spacer graft is inserted between the inferior border of the tarsus and the recessed edge of the retractors.

roid, and the limits this places on the predictability of the surgery. Careful discussion with the patient and use of the correct procedure will minimize postoperative complications and maximize patient satisfaction.

REFERENCES

1. Sergott RC, Glaser JS: Graves Ophthalmopathy, A Clinical and Immunological Review, Surv Ophthalmol 26:1 1981.

2. Waller RR: Eyelid Malposition in Graves Ophthalmopathy. Trans Am Ophthalmol Soc 80:855, 1982.

3. Gay AJ, Wolkstein MA: Topical Guanethidine Therapy for Endocrine Lid Retraction, Arch Ophthalmol 76:365, 1966.

4. Waller RR: Eyelid Malposition in Graves Ophthalmopathy. Trans Am Ophthalmol Soc 80:855, 1982.

5. Goldstein I: Recession of the Levator Muscle for Lagophthalmos in Exophthalmos Goiter, Arch Ophthalmol 1:389, 1934.

6. Dryden RM: Scleral Grafting for Upper Eyelid Retraction. In Symposium on Surgical Management of Thyroid Ophthalmopathy, Proceedings of the Annual Meeting of the American Academy of Ophthalmology. Chicago, 1980.

5

BLEPHAROPTOSIS

Any time the eyelid droops, blepharoptosis results. The condition is cosmetically noticeable even in the earliest stages. When a significant visual field defect occurs, it becomes a functional problem. Blepharoptosis repair is one of the most common oculoplastic procedures performed. The appropriate evaluation of the patient with blepharoptosis will lead the surgeon to choose an appropriate surgical procedure and minimize the incidence of complications. An understanding of the etiology of the various subtypes of eyelid ptosis is also important in surgical decision making.

ETIOLOGY

The etiology of blepharoptosis can be divided into five main categories: aponeurotic, muscular, neurological, traumatic, and mechanical. The terms "acquired" and "congenital" can be misleading and should be avoided. Although most cases of acquired ptosis are aponeurotic, not all are. Likewise, although most cases of congenital ptosis are muscular, some may be neurological or aponeurotic. Using the proper terminology leads to less confusion. Determining the subtype of ptosis leads to choosing the proper surgical procedure.

The most common etiology of blepharoptosis is aponeurotic. This condition is typically seen as adult acquired ptosis but may occur congenitally or through trauma. The levator aponeurosis is either stretched or detached from its insertion on the tarsus.

Muscular ptosis occurs when there is a replacement of striated muscle fibers with noncontractile fibrous tissue. Typically the worse the ptosis, the less normal muscle is found microscopically. This condition is unilateral in 75% of patients and is the most common type of congenital ptosis seen.

Various etiologies of neurological ptosis are encountered. Some of the more common are trauma, myasthenia gravis, myotonic dystrophy, and chronic progressive external ophthalmoplegia (CPEO). In myasthenia gravis there is a defect in neuromuscular communication that occurs at the junction between the neuron and the muscle fiber. This is due to antibodies to acetylcholine receptors of the muscle end plate. Myotonic dystrophy is an autosomal dominant form of muscular dystrophy. In CPEO a gradual deterioration in extraocular muscle function is seen secondary to mitochondrial dysfunction.

Traumatic ptosis may not deserve its own category. In reality most cases of traumatic ptosis are either aponeurotic or neurologic in origin. Mechanical blepharoptosis is seen whenever a mass or swelling of the eyelid causes it to droop. Tumor, trauma, edema, poor lymphatic outflow, and other etiologies could be responsible for such drooping.

PREOPERATIVE EVALUATION

The evaluation of the patient with blepharoptosis has several goals. It should help identify the type of ptosis the patient has and indicate which particular operation is appropriate. Additionally, it should identify any preexisting conditions that might call for modifications of surgical goals or even the abandonment of the surgical plan. In other words, a detailed evaluation should keep the surgeon and patient out of trouble.

The actual amount of ptosis is determined by measuring the MRD_1. The patient is asked to look directly at a small light source. The ipsilateral frontalis muscle is suppressed and the contralateral eyelid is elevated if it is ptotic. This suppresses the contribution of the frontalis muscle and Herring's law to eyelid height. The distance, in millimeters, between the light reflex on the central cornea and the central eyelid margin is the MRD_1. Negative measurements are possible. Normal values are between 3.5 and 5 mm.

The Burke levator function (BLF) measures the eyelid excursion from maximum downgaze to maximum upgaze. The ipsilateral frontalis muscle is suppressed by placing several fingers on the eyebrow. This is arguably the most important measurement in ptosis evaluation. Normal values are between 15 and 18 mm.

The vertical fissure width in downgaze is measured in maximal downgaze. Normally the levator aponeurosis acts as a check ligament in downgaze, keeping the eyelid from closing with reading. Normal measurements are between 2 and 4 mm.

Ductions and versions of the eyes are evaluated. Deficiencies in these can point to unusual conditions such as third nerve palsies, CPEO, and double-elevator palsies.

The presence of strabismus is important to note. If present, it prompts a decision whether to correct the strabismus and if so whether correction should precede ptosis surgery. Correction of vertical misalignments can have a profound effect on eyelid position and, if they are going to be corrected, they should be corrected first.

Various danger signs are evaluated. Lagophthalmos, the inability to completely close the eyelid with *gentle* closure, is measured. This mimics what occurs when the patient is sleeping. Corneal staining, Bell's phenomenon, and dry eye are also looked for. A basic secretor test or other indicators of a dry eye condition are very important. The presence of any of these danger signs is notable and may cause a modification of the surgical goals for the patient (i.e., placing the eyelid lower than would otherwise be optimal). The presence of several of these could be a reason to not perform the desired surgery.

In patients with good levator function a Neo-synephrine test can be employed. Several drops of 10% phenylephrine hydrochloride (Neosynephrine, Sanofi Pharmaceuticals, New York) are placed under the eyelid. The maximum height of the eyelid is measured as an MRD_1. The maximum height typically takes several minutes to occur. If a significant response to Neosynephrine is seen, this is an indication that a conjunctival–Müller's muscle resection procedure may be useful.

In patients with poor levator function, an MLD measurement is used. This will help determine how much levator resection should be performed. The patient is asked to gaze maximally upward. The distance from the inferior limbus to the upper eyelid margin is measured in millimeters. A normal measurement is 9 mm. Negative measurements are possible.

The position of the eyelid crease is recorded. Normally this is between 7 and 10 mm above the eyelid border. In aponeurotic ptosis this is often increased. In muscular ptosis it is unchanged or absent (owing to poor muscle development).

An approximation of orbicularis strength can be made. This is important when the ptosis is due to neurological causes. Poor orbicularis strength is often seen with myotonic dystrophy and can lead to lagophthalmos and corneal problems postoperatively.

If myasthenia gravis is suspected, a fatigue test and/or Tensilon test (edrophonium chloride, ICN Pharmaceuticals, Costa Mesa, CA) should be performed. Alternatively the patient can be referred to a neuro-ophthalmologist for evaluation.

History is very important. Systemic disease can cause eyelid ptosis. The age at onset of the ptosis as well as other symptoms occurring should be sought. It is important to remember that not all ptosis occurring at birth is muscular in origin. Likewise, a 60-year-old patient with no history of surgery may have decided only recently to investigate the possibility of surgical correction of a muscular ptosis present since birth.

SURGICAL DECISION MAKING

The most important factors in differentiating aponeurotic from muscular ptosis are history, Burke levator function, eyelid crease position, and fissure width in downgaze (see Table 5-1). In aponeurotic ptosis the patient will typically have good levator function (between 12 and 18 mm). The history is that of gradual onset beginning in middle to later life. The eyelid crease is characteristically elevated. Since the levator muscle is stretched or detached, it does not perform the function of a check ligament in downgaze, and the fissure width in downgaze is narrowed and sometimes actually closed (Table 5-1).

Muscular ptosis will have moderate to poor levator function of between 0 and 10 mm. The history is that of a ptosis essentially stable since birth. The eyelid crease is either in a normal position or is absent in severe cases. Owing to the fibrotic, inelastic nature of the levator muscle, the fissure width in downgaze is often increased.

When dealing with an aponeurotic ptosis, either a conjunctival–Müller's muscle resection or a levator advancement procedure is employed. If the patient responded to the Neosynephrine test and does not need skin resection, a conjunctival–Müller's muscle procedure is a reasonable choice. The Neosynephrine test dictates the amount of resection to be performed. The range of resection is between 6.5 and 9.0 mm. When the ptotic lid rises to a height equal to the normal lid, an 8 mm resection is performed. If the lid rises above the normal lid, a decreased amount of resection is performed, with 6.5 mm being the minimum. If the lid rises, but not to the desired height, the amount of resection is increased up to a maximum of 9.0 mm. If no response is seen with the Neosynephrine test, the conjunctival–Müller's muscle resection should not be employed.

TABLE 5-1. Factors distinguishing aponeurotic from muscular ptosis

	History	Levator function	Crease position	Fissure width in downgaze
Aponeurotic ptosis	Gradual onset, middle age or older	≥12 mm	Often elevated	Decreased
Muscular ptosis	Stable, present at birth	≤10 mm	Normal or absent	Increased

A levator advancement procedure can be employed in all cases of aponeurotic ptosis. It is especially useful when skin excision is desired. The amount of advancement is determined intraoperatively by sitting the patient up and judging the eyelid height and contour.

A muscular ptosis is corrected by either levator advancement or a frontalis sling procedure. The main determinant is the levator function. If the levator function is 4 mm or greater, a levator resection should be used. If the levator function is 3 mm or less, a frontalis sling is employed. In most cases a sling of fascia lata is recommended, as the long-term results are the best.

The MLD formula is utilized to determine the amount of levator resection performed. If the ptosis is bilateral, the number of millimeters of resection is found by subtracting $MLD_{ptotic\ lid}$ from 9 and multiplying by 3. If only one eyelid is involved and the plan is to match the ptotic eyelids height to that of the normal eyelid the amount of resection found as follows: $(MLD_{normal\ lid} - MLD_{ptotic\ lid})3$. For example, if the MLD of the normal eyelid is 8 mm and that of the ptotic eyelid is 2 mm, the formula dictates a resection of 18 mm.

If a frontalis sling is performed, the lid height is set intraoperatively. The lid is placed at or just above the desired final position.

A neurologic ptosis is corrected by utilizing levator advancement, levator resection, or a frontalis sling. The decision is made primarily on the basis of the levator function. In myasthenia gravis it is often advisable to perform a sling procedure even when the levator function would suggest performing levator advancement. This is due to the variable nature of the levator function in myasthenia gravis, and the patient can use the frontalis muscle to varying degrees to compensate. In certain conditions with poor orbicularis strength, such as myotonic dystrophy, it is advisable to utilize a silicone rod sling instead of fascia lata. This type of sling stretches, allowing better closure of the eyelids, protecting the cornea better, and minimizing problems related to exposure.

SURGICAL TECHNIQUES

Müller's Muscle–Conjunctival Resection

After the patient is sedated, a frontal nerve block is placed just lateral to the supraorbital grove with a 25 gauge, 1.5 inch needle. An equal mixture of 0.5% bupivicaine hydrochloride (Marcaine, Astra Pharmaceutical, L.P., Wayne, PA) and 2% lidocaine hydrochloride (Xylocaine, Astra Pharmaceutical) is used. A 4-0 silk traction suture is place centrally just above the lashes, and a Desmarres retractor is used to evert the lid. The predetermined amount of Müller's muscle resection is marked with a 6-0 silk suture passed just through conjunctiva (Figure 5-1). Bleeding from Müller's muscle can occur if a deeper pass is made. Bites are taken medially, centrally, and temporally. A forceps grasps both conjunctiva and the Müller's muscle and loosens the muscle from the overlying levator aponeurosis. A Putterman Müller's muscle resection clamp is placed between the marking suture and the superior tarsal border. The clamp is closed and contains only conjunctiva and Müller's muscle (Figure 5-2). A 5-0 double-armed plain gut suture is placed 1.5 mm below the clamp as a running horizontal mattress suture Figure 5-3). A #15 blade is used to remove the tissue in the clamp. Maintaining a "metal-on-metal" feel

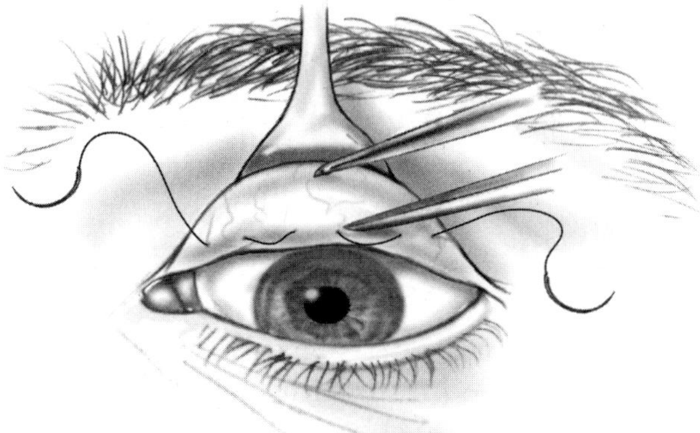

FIGURE 5-1. A marking suture is placed a predetermined distance form the superior tarsal border.

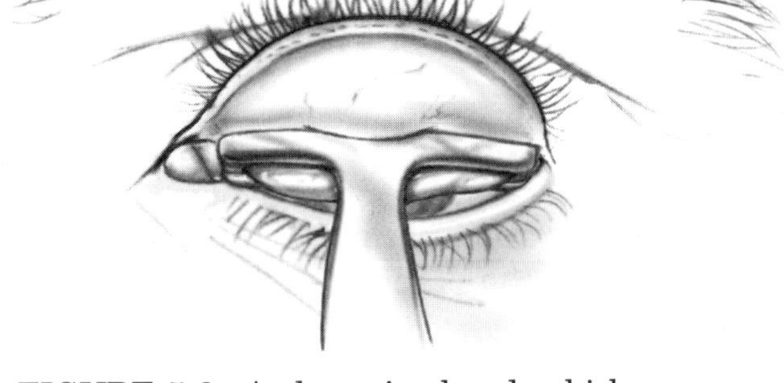

FIGURE 5-2. A clamp is placed, which now contains conjunctiva and Müller's muscle.

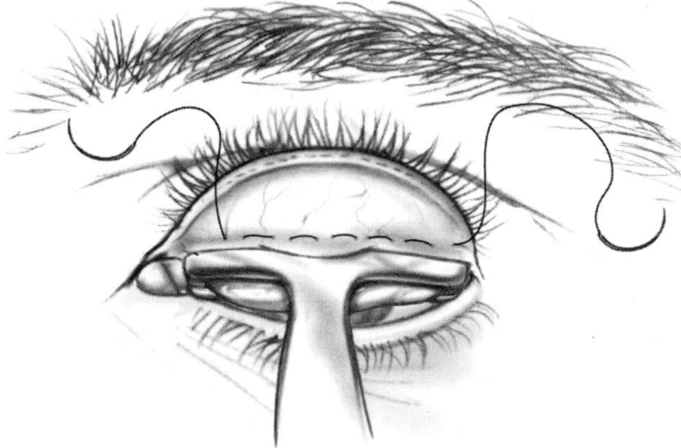

FIGURE 5-3. A 5-0 plain gut suture is placed superior to the clamp in a running mattress fashion.

between clamp and blade will help prevent cutting the suture (Figure 5-4). The needles are passed full thickness through the lid, exiting on the skin. A small piece of surgical tape holds the suture in place. A mild pressure dressing is placed for 24 hours. In one week the surgical tape is removed and suture ends trimmed if necessary.

Levator Aponeurosis Advancement

An eyelid crease incision is marked. When skin resection is desired, this is marked utilizing the pinch technique to minimize the risk of lagophthalmos. An equal mixture of 0.5 % Marcaine and 2% Xylocaine, both with epinephrine, is injected in the marked area. A small amount of anesthetic is used to prevent distortion of the eyelid and to avoid complicating the intraoperative assessment of eyelid height. The incision is made with a #15 blade, and a skin muscle flap is removed with Westcott scissors. In the area overlying the cornea, an inferior skin muscle flap is dissected for 5 mm, exposing the tarsus.

When the lid is pulled downward, the edge of levator aponeurosis is often visible just deep to the orbital fat. The edge of the aponeurosis or the tissue just deep to the orbital fat is grasped and pulled inferiorly. The tissue just anterior to this is pulled perpendicularly outward. Westcott scissors cut the tissue between the forceps, staying parallel to the plane of the aponeurosis (Figure 5-5). This avoids

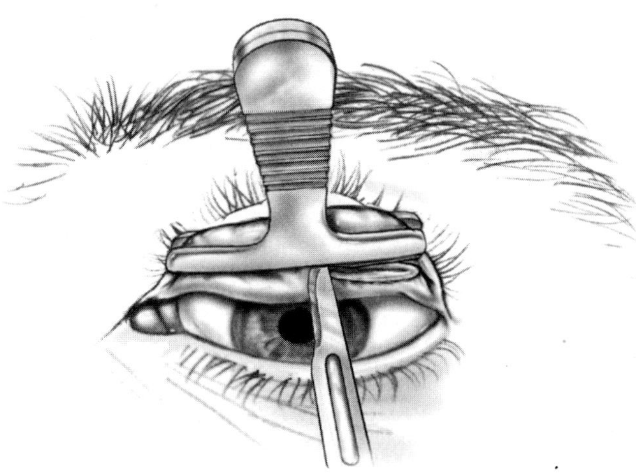

FIGURE 5-4. The tissue within the clamp is removed with the blade, maintaining a metal-on-metal feel to minimize the chances of cutting the suture.

FIGURE 5-5. Westcott scissors are used to incise the orbital septum.

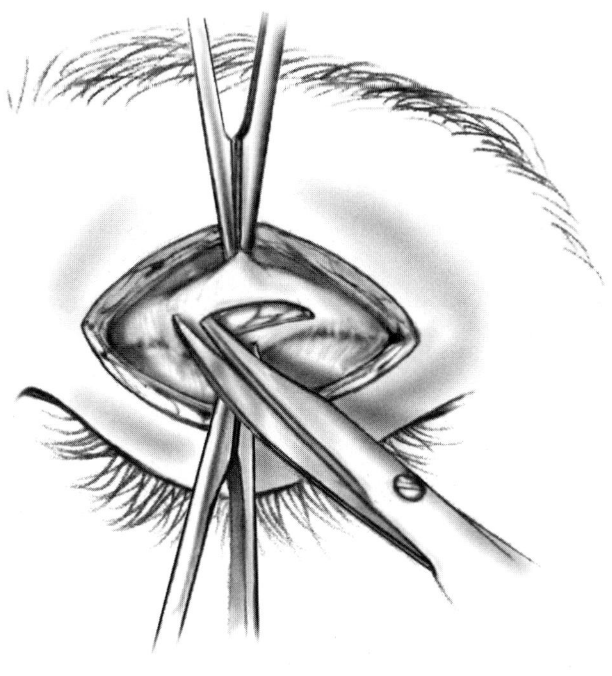

damage to the aponeurosis. The levator aponeurosis is exposed and separated from the orbital septum (Figure 5-6). This is crucial because incorporating the septum in the advancement would lead to lagophthalmos. Just below the superior tarsal border, a 6-0 silk or 5-0 poly(butyl ester) (Novafil) suture is passed partial thickness through the tarsus for a distance of about 5 mm. (Figure 5-7) The lid is everted to be certain the suture has not penetrated through full-thickness tarsus. The suture is placed in a mattress fashion through

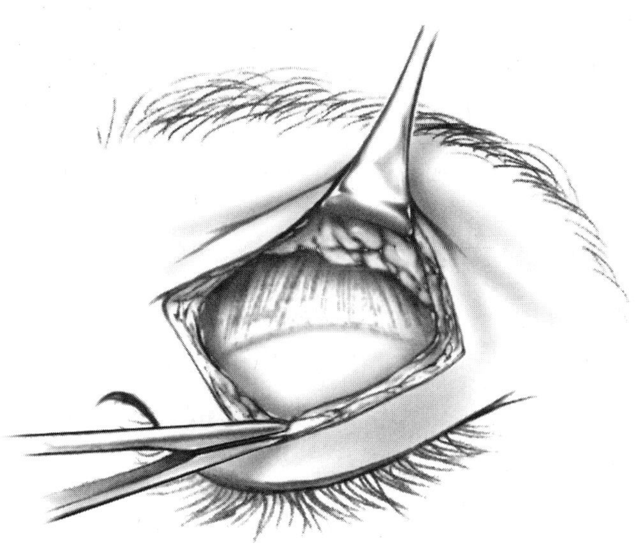

FIGURE 5-6. The levator aponeurosis is seen to be slightly dehisced from the tarsus.

FIGURE 5-7. A suture is placed through partial thickness tarsus.

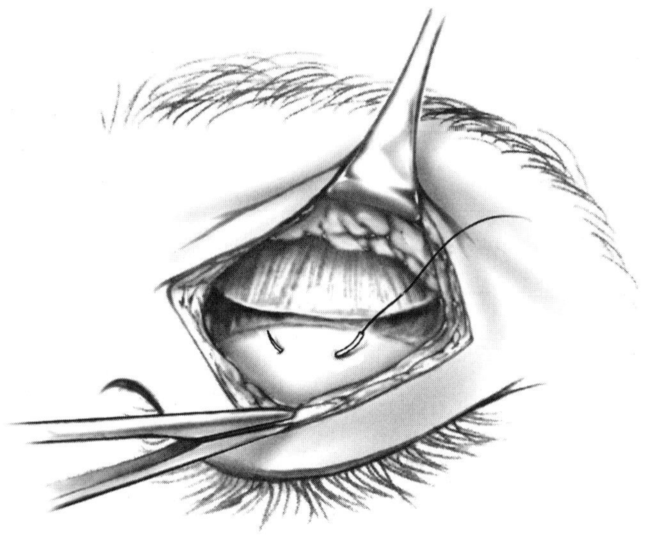

the levator aponeurosis and tied temporarily (Figure 5-8). A piece of 4-0 silk suture approximately 6 inches long can be placed under the throw of 6-0 silk. This knot-releasing suture can be pulled upward to loosen the mattress suture when adjustments are made; it is removed prior to final tying of the mattress suture. The patient is brought to a sitting position and asked to open the eyes; a slight overcorrection of about 1 mm is desirable on the table (Figure 5-9). The suture can be loosened or tightened or a larger bite of aponeurosis taken until the appropriate lid height is achieved. Medial and lateral sutures can be placed if the eyelid contour needs to be adjusted. The patient is returned to a supine position and the suture tied. Skin closure is with a 6-0 polypropylene (Prolene) running subcutaneous suture. For the next 48 hours, ice is applied for 15 minutes every hour the patient is awake. Mastisol and surgical tape are placed over the wound. Sutures are removed in one week.

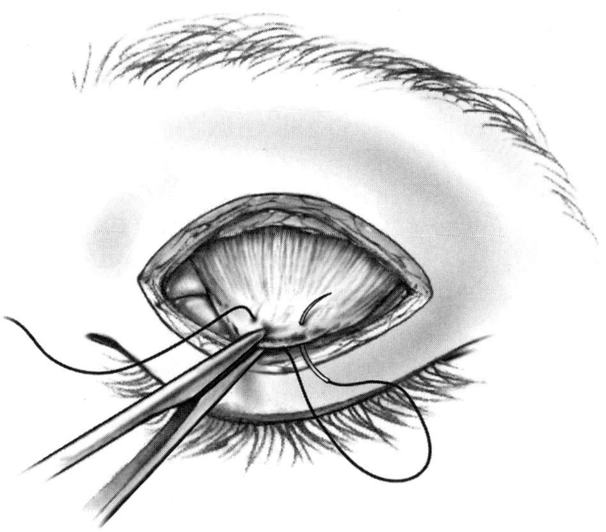

FIGURE 5-8. Both arms of the suture are passed through the edge of the levator aponeurosis.

FIGURE 5-9. With the patient sitting up and fully awake, the eyelid height is judged.

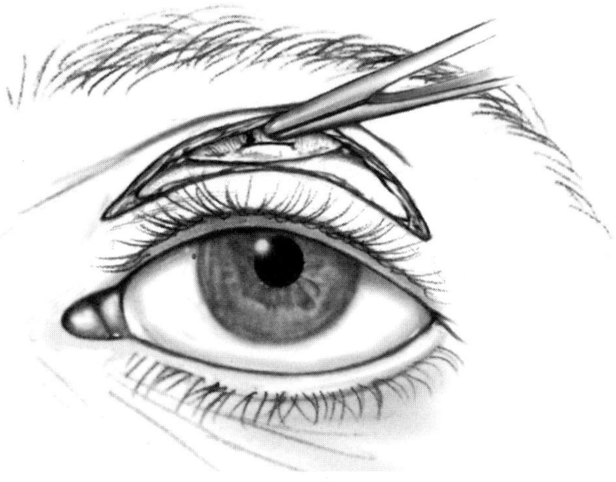

Levator Resection

Depending on the age of the patient, either general or local anesthesia can be used. The eyelid crease is marked and an infiltration of an equal mixture of 0.5% Marcaine and 2% Xylocaine, both with epinephrine, is given. An incision is made with a #15 blade through the skin and orbicularis muscle. Westcott scissors are used to dissect through the orbital septum (Figure 5-10), exposing the underlying levator muscle. Westcott scissors tent the conjunctiva, Müller's muscle, and levator muscle upward at the superior tarsal border at the far medial border of the tarsus. A #15 blade cuts through these tissues. The same incision is made at the far temporal end of the tarsus (Figure 5-11). A Putterman ptosis clamp is placed just above the tarsus. This clamp holds the levator muscle, Müller's muscle, and conjunctiva. A #15 blade is used to separate these tissues from the superior tarsal border. Vertical incisions through these tissues are made at the medial and temporal ends of the clamp. The conjunctiva is dis-

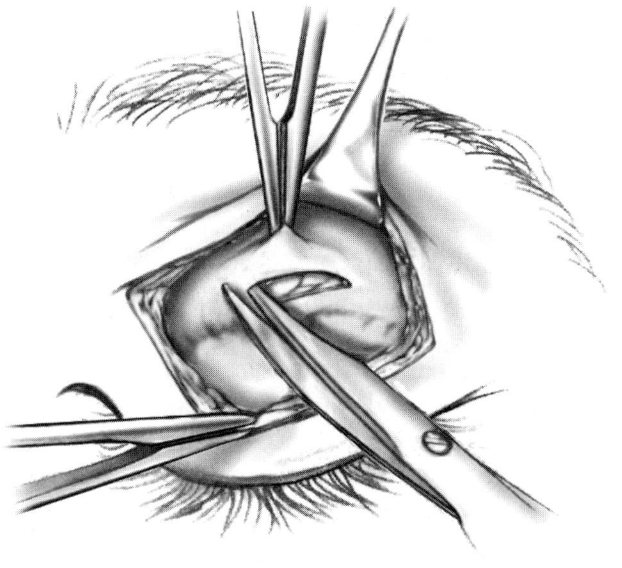

FIGURE 5-10. The orbital septum is opened and the levator aponeurosis is exposed.

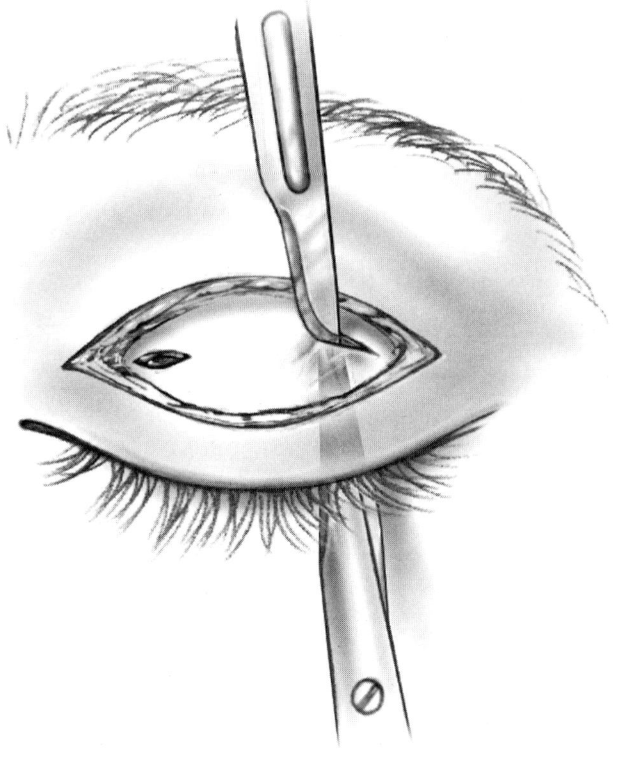

FIGURE 5-11. A Westcott scissors pushes upward at the superior tarsal border, and a blade is used to make a buttonhole through conjunctiva, Müller's muscle, and the levator aponeurosis.

sected free from the underside of Müller's muscle (Figure 5-12) and reattached to the superior tarsal border with a running 6-0 plain gut suture. Superior dissection through Müller's muscle and levator muscle is carried out medially and temporally (Figure 5-13). These lines of dissection should not converge, since this would produce unpredictable results. How far the dissection proceeds superiorly depends on the amount of levator resection planned. It is important not to cut the horns of the levator. Avoid reaching far superiorly with the scissors. Small superior cuts, on alternating sides of the levator, will deliver the muscle to the surgeon and not sever the levator horns. A strip of orbicular muscle is removed from the superior tarsal border. A double-armed 6-0 polyglactin 910 (Vicryl) suture is passed partial thickness through the central tarsus, several millimeters below the superior border. It is then passed in mattress fashion through the levator muscle at the predetermined position. This suture is temporarily tied and the eyelid height checked. If acceptable, the suture is temporarily loosened to allow easier placement of the remaining sutures. Medial and lateral sutures of the same type are placed, utilizing the same amount of resection as with the central suture. The central suture is tied first. The medial and lateral sutures are tem-

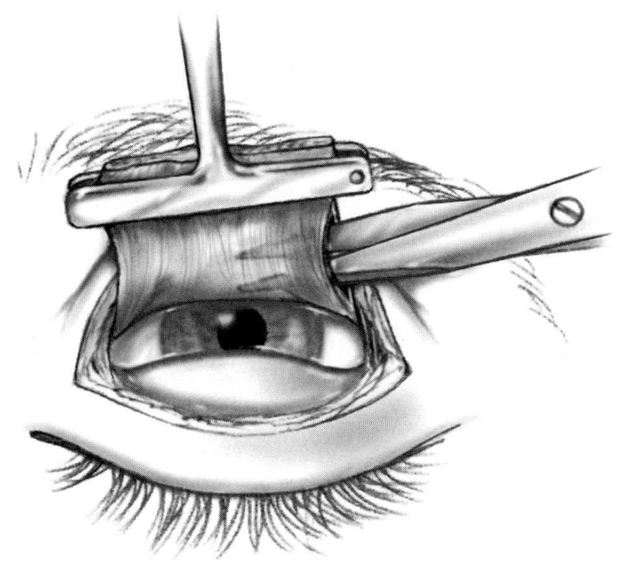

FIGURE 5-12. The conjunctiva is dissected from the levator aponeurosis.

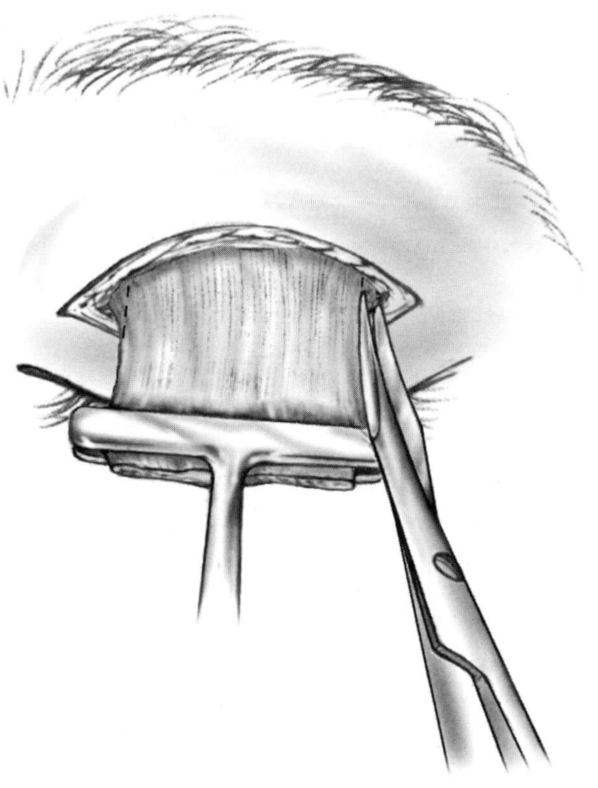

FIGURE 5-13. A superior dissection through Müller's muscle and the levator aponeurosis is performed medially and laterally.

porarily tied (Figure 5-14). These sutures affect the contour of the lid, and the amount of resection can be varied to achieve an acceptable eyelid contour. Once appropriate medial and lateral contours have been achieved, the sutures are tied permanently. The advanced levator and Müller's muscle are clamped with a hemostat and excised. Running or interrupted 6-0 Prolene or 6-0 plain sutures are placed closing the skin. The running 6-0 Prolene suture can be placed in a subcutaneous fashion. Three deep bites incorporating the skin edges and the advanced edge of the levator muscle are taken to re-form the eyelid crease. These are placed prior to final skin closure. Ointment is placed in the eye and a mild pressure patch placed for 24 hours. Sutures are removed in one week when appropriate.

Frontalis Sling

General or local anesthesia is used depending on the age of the patient. A single rhomboid pattern is marked. Just above the lash border, two incisions are marked, each about 3 mm long. The incisions are centered approximately 6 mm medial and temporal to the point directly above the central cornea. The desired positions can be checked and adjusted by placing cotton-tipped applicators under each mark and elevating the eyelid. Three eyebrow incisions are used. The central incision is directly above the central cornea. The medial and lateral brow incisions are marked just medial and lateral to their respective lid incisions. An injection of an equal mixture of 0.5% Marcaine and 2% Xylocaine, both with epinephrine, is given. Small incisions are made in the brow and eyelid area through skin and muscle. A small inferior dissection deep to frontalis muscle is made through the central brow incision. This will allow the fascia lata knot to be buried easily. The supraorbital nerve can be damaged if the medial brow incision is too deep. A Wright fascia needle is used to pass a piece of fascia lata 2 mm wide and 15 cm long. The needle is passed from the temporal eyebrow incision to the temporal eyelid incision. The needle passes under the orbicularis, staying above the septum. It is important to always know where the globe is with respect to the needle. The fascia is passed through the eye of the needle and withdrawn (Figure 5-15). The same technique is used to pass the fascia from the temporal eyelid incision to the medial eyelid incision. The plane of passage is just above the tarsal plate. The fascia is then passed from the medial eyelid incision to the medial eyebrow incision. The fascia from the medial and temporal eyebrow incisions is

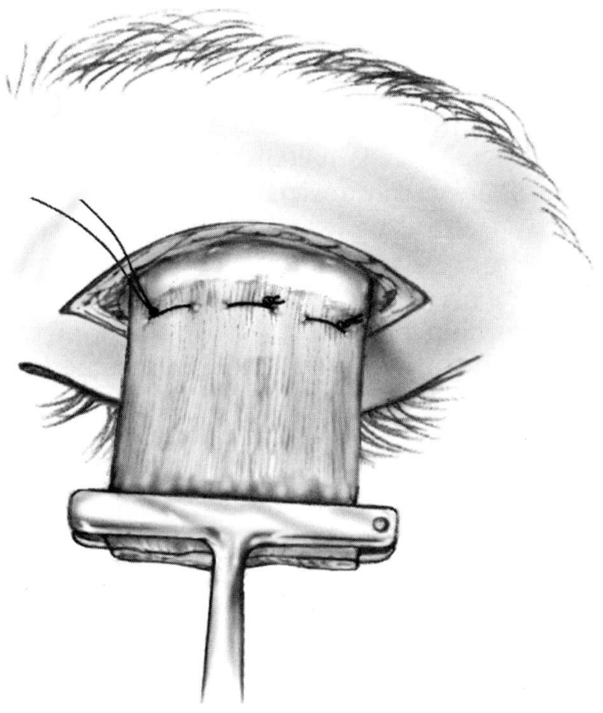

FIGURE 5-14. To control the height and contour of the eyelid, three sutures are placed through the predetermined amount of levator aponeurosis.

FIGURE 5-15. Fascia lata is passed with a Wright fascia needle from the temporal eyelid incision the temporal eyebrow incision.

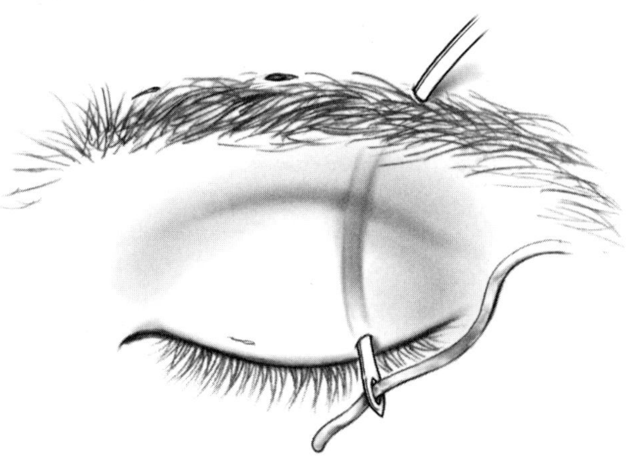

passed to the central eyebrow incision (Figure 5-16). A piece of 6-0 Vicryl suture is placed under the fascia lata. The fascia is tied with the first throw of a simple square knot. A patient who is awake should be brought to a sitting position to judge the eyelid height. A slight overcorrection is desirable. If the patient is asleep, the height is adjusted until the lid is at or just above the desired position. It is important to tuck the temporarily tied fascia lata knot into the previously created subfrontalis pocket prior to judging the eyelid height. Once an adequate height and contour are achieved, the Vicryl suture is tied around the fascia lata to help prevent early slippage of the knot. The final throw of the fascia lata square knot is tied (Figure 5-17), and the knot is buried in the central incision. Several 6-0 plain sutures are used to close the incisions. Ointment is placed in the eye and a mild pressure patch is used to close the eye for 24 hours. Ocular lubrication, especially at night, is important to avoid corneal complications in the early postoperative period.

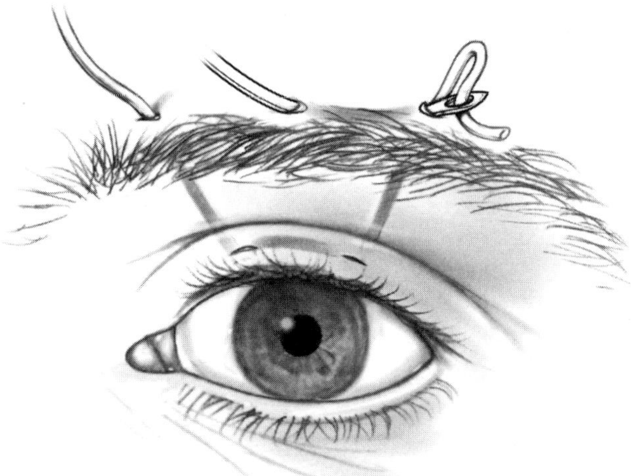

FIGURE 5-16. The fascia lata is passed from the medial and temporal eyebrow incision to the middle eyebrow incision.

FIGURE 5-17. A simple square knot is tied in the fascia lata. A Vicryl suture is tied around the knot, helping to secure it.

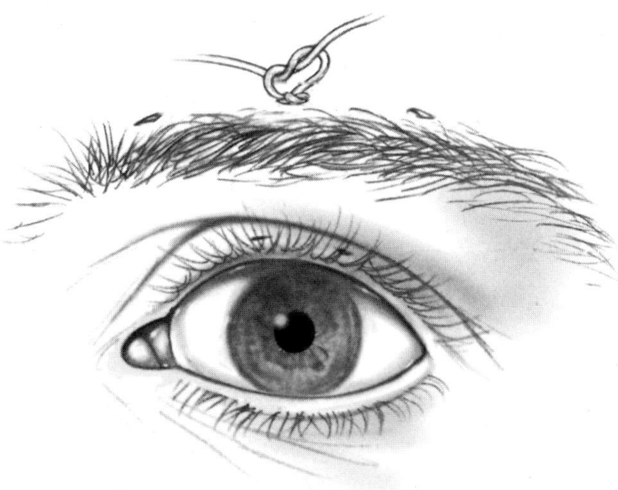

6

EYELID RECONSTRUCTION

ETIOLOGY

Description of Disorder

Eyelid defects require precise closure to maintain proper function and appearance of the eye. Repair of the defects depends on their location and extent. Superficial tissue involving the skin and orbicularis may require simple closure or development of flaps or grafts. Full-thickness eyelid injury requires precise assessment of available surrounding tissue and closure of the lid at several levels. Deeper injury to the orbit may involve exploration and repair of the lacrimal drainage system, orbital bones, or the globe itself. Evaluation and repair of these delicate structures requires a fundamental knowledge of the regional anatomy as well as a thorough understanding of reconstructive techniques.

Among the most common eyelid deficits encountered by ophthalmic plastic surgeons are those that are full thickness. Simple vertical full-thickness lacerations without canalicular involvement can be closed with the classic "three-suture" method. Lacerations that involve loss of tissue present greater challenges. Numerous reconstructive techniques, which depend not only on the extent of the defect but also on the quality and availability of surrounding tissue, exist to repair the tissue deficits.

Prevalence and Significance of Disorder

Eyelid defects are usually caused by trauma or surgery to remove tumors. The resulting defect may be loss of a small amount of superficial tissue, or absence of an entire eyelid. Removal of small eyelid margin masses usually allows the surgeon to prepare a pentagonal wedge defect with even borders. However, large lesions as well as malignant neoplasms that are excised using Mohs micrographic surgery often present with large defects and irregular borders.

Repair may be more difficult in certain individuals with preexisting medical conditions. Those with prior radiation exposure or other skin disorders may have significant tissue shrinkage or destruction at different levels of the skin. For example, full-thickness tissue scarring may be present following radiation exposure or herpes zoster dermatitis. Anterior lamellar defects, primarily of the skin, are present in numerous dermatologic conditions, including numerous types of dermatitis and many connective tissue disorders. Another important consideration is that certain reconstructive procedures have limited success in particular patients. For example, individuals who have received radiation treatment may not accept free grafts (skin or other autogenous material).

Skin quality and laxity differ among patients. Those with excess skin and "loose" eyelids with significant canthal laxity tend to be older patients, who will have more available tissue than typical younger patients. With more available tissue, repair of the eyelid defect usually involves a less complicated repair. Patients with prior eyelid surgery, burns, or radiation tend to have less lax and mobile eyelids. Also, individuals with dermatologic conditions that limit skin elasticity or mobility may require more complex reconstruction.

Subtypes

Congenital colobomas involve full-thickness loss of part of an eyelid, usually the upper. These rare defects often result in no functional impairment, and significant keratopathy seldom develops. Congenital colobomas may present with a rounded superior border that contains a small amount of normal tarsus. This residual tarsus should be removed during the reconstructive process to allow proper tissue apposition, and to avoid a raised tissue deformity at the superior wound margin. Repair of most colobomas can be initiated if signs or symptoms of corneal exposure develop. Most surgeons prefer to delay treatment until at least 6 months.

Full-thickness traumatic defects are much more common than congenital defects. Frequently, lacerations that appear to involve a small region of the eyelid skin are associated with a large vertical tear of the tarsal plate. Lacerations may be perpendicular to the lid margin, or they may be irregular and highly angulated. Traumatic defects often involve situations where all tissue is present but may be difficult to locate or identify. When a significant amount of tissue is absent or severely damaged, flaps must be created and mobilized.

Repair of the canalicular system may be required in conjunction with eyelid repair when trauma results in lacerations in the area of during extirpation of tumors. Lacerations of the canalicular system involve a common subtype of eyelid trauma. The lacrimal drainage system must be inspected in all situations when trauma to this area is suspected. Canalicular trauma may be caused by direct as well as indirect trauma. The drainage system should be inspected visually, and canalicular probing and irrigation performed before repair is initiated. An experienced surgeon should perform the repair within several days of the injury. While most patients with a single functioning canaliculus are asymptomatic, some may have epiphora.

When surgery is planned in the area of the canaliculi, the surgeon should consider placing a Bowman probe in the canaliculi prior to initiating the procedure. The probe will allow the surgeon to judge the location of the lacrimal system and thus avoid unnecessary injury to the canaliculi.

Pathophysiology

Proper eyelid reconstruction requires thorough preoperative evaluation of the involved structures. The surgeon should consider the integrity and relationships of the five basic eyelid components: anterior lamella (skin and orbicularis), posterior lamella (tarsus and conjunctiva), canthal tendons, canaliculi, and levator muscle.

Eyelid skin, primarily because of its attenuated dermis, is the thinnest skin of the body. While this characteristic allows for rapid healing of incisions, it also creates difficulty for the surgeon attempting to find a suitable donor area for skin graft with appropriate color, texture, and thickness. Common donor areas in eyelid reconstruction are other eyelid skin and pre- and postauricular skin. Full-thickness skin grafts are commonly utilized in eyelid surgery, either alone or in conjunction with flaps, to repair small defects ranging from approximately 1 to 5 cm. A full-thickness skin graft includes the two layers of skin, epidermis and dermis, along with a small amount of subdermal fat.

Eyelid skin, particularly from the contralateral lid, tends to be the best match for eyelid defects. Upper eyelid skin always provides the best match for the contralateral upper eyelid. The second choice of donor tissue is usually any eyelid skin. For some patients, particularly young individuals or those in whom large areas require repair, adequate eyelid skin may not be available. The preferred donor site for eyelids is generally the postauricular sulcus, the skin of which heals well in the periorbital region. Postauricular skin may provide an excellent match, based on its greater thickness, for grafts to the lower eyelid. Thicker donor tissue from the preauricular and supraclavicular regions provides appropriate donor tissue to repair defects outside the periorbital region. Multiple grafts may be required to repair a large defect.

The medial and lateral canthal ligaments provide structural support to the orbicularis muscle by connecting the tarsus to the periosteum of the orbital bone. Fibers from the medial canthal ligament insert on both the anterior and posterior lacrimal crest. The deep fibers that insert on the posterior lacrimal crest serve as the anterior border of the deep pretarsal orbicularis muscles and also as a posterior anchor. Successful reconstructive surgery in the medial canthal area requires reestablishment of this important relationship.

The lateral canthal ligament is composed primarily of fibrous strands continuous with the upper and lower tarsus. The lateral canthal ligament inserts just inside the lateral orbital rim at Whitnall's lateral orbital tubercle. In lower eyelid reconstruction, the surgeon must recognize the posterior direction of this ligament. The lateral canthal angle, formed by the union of the upper and lower eyelids, rests approximately 2 mm higher than the medial canthal angle.

The surgeon should consider the integrity of the lacrimal drainage system following eyelid trauma. The puncta in the upper and lower eyelids are 8 and 10 mm lateral to the tear sac, respectively. If trauma occurs medial to this point, there is a higher probability of damage to the lacrimal system. The canaliculi are buried

Eyelid Reconstruction

within the orbicularis muscle. The canaliculi are vertical for the initial 2 mm, before each becomes horizontal at a right angle dilation termed the ampulla.

The levator muscle is the primary elevator of the upper eyelid. Following trauma, the levator may become disinserted from the tarsus. This dehiscence, which may be detected by recognizing the white aponeurosis that retracts on attempted upgaze, should be repaired.

Reconstruction of eyelid defects requires adherence to basic surgical principles. If adequate tissue is not available for direct closure, repair will involve mobilizing local tissue or providing graft material. For full-thickness eyelid repair, the two main layers, the anterior and posterior lamellae, must be preserved. Free grafts can be used to supplement either the anterior or posterior lamella, but separate free grafts should not be used to reconstruct a single full-thickness eyelid. However, a single composite (full-thickness) graft from the contralateral lid donor site may be used.

CLINICAL EVALUATION

History

While the immediate cause of an eyelid defect is usually not difficult to elicit, several circumstances can determine how the preoperative evaluation proceeds. Following trauma, the mechanism of injury can determine the depth of the wound and whether a foreign body is present. Decreased visual acuity can suggest an injury to the globe or optic nerve. Orbital fractures may be associated with diplopia, hypesthesia, abnormal globe position, epistaxis, or pain during eye or jaw movement. If the injury is caused by an animal bite, the rabies immunization status of the animal should be determined. If the wound follows removal of a tumor, the surgeon should confirm that all margins are free of tumor.

A history of injury or surgery to the eyelids should be elicited. Patients with prior surgery or trauma may have atypical anatomic landmarks. The patient should be asked about any irregular wound healing that has taken place in the past. A history of any prior ocular injury should be determined, along with known allergies and a list of medications.

Examination

A thorough ophthalmologic examination should be performed on all patients with ocular or orbital trauma. Often a wound appears to be superficial, but examination reveals a deeper track into the orbit or eye. When a laceration occurs to the eyelids, it is often easily recognized. However, concurrent blunt trauma may cause additional fractures, tendon and other soft tissue injuries, and numerous intraocular defects. The surgeon should perform a full evaluation of the eye, followed by inspection of the surrounding soft tissue adnexa, orbit, and face.

The examination should begin with evaluation of the eye. Visual acuity, pupillary response, and intraocular pressure should be checked. Slitlamp and dilated fundus examinations should be completed. Eyelid edema and patient discomfort may limit surgeon's ability to assess the globe, and evaluation may need to be repeated as the tissue heals.

Evaluation of the soft tissue adnexa should confirm the depth and extent of lacerations. If the lid margin is involved, the posterior lamella should also be inspected and the length of the laceration documented. Eyelid position and function should be examined, although edema and discomfort may limit the surgeon's ability to assess levator function. If fat appears within the depths of a wound, the surgeon can assume that the septum has been violated, and there is a higher possibility that the orbit is involved.

The canalicular system should be closely examined for laceration in the vicinity. If a laceration is present, often the severed canaliculus can be viewed. If there is any doubt about whether the canaliculus has been severed, the system should be probed and irrigated. Even if there is a suggestion of blunt trauma to the area, probing and irrigation are appropriate to assess the continuity of the lacrimal system.

Displacement or "rounding" of the canthal angles suggests injury to the canthal tendons. If the medial canthus is displaced, there is a greater incidence of canalicular injury. Lateral displacement of the punctum is another sign of canalicular damage.

Orbital examination involves assessing extraocular muscle function in all fields of gaze. Hypesthesia of the cheek should be tested. The orbital rim should be palpated to detect a bony deformity. Proptosis and significant tightness of the eyelids may indicate orbital hemorrhage. Abnormal globe position (particularly hypophthalmos) may indicate a fracture. Pain upon chewing or opening the mouth, or depression of the malar eminence of the cheek, may be associated with a zygomatic fracture. If fracture or foreign body is suspected, a CT scan with direct axial and coronal views with 3 mm cuts should be obtained prior to eyelid reconstruction.

Diagnostic Testing

Following appropriate examination, the surgeon determines the extent of the eyelid defect. If only the anterior lamella is injured, appropriate repair may include simple closure, harvesting and placement of a skin graft, or mobilization of a skin flap. For a full-thickness laceration with minimal or no tissue loss, direct closure with the classic three-suture technique should be attempted. For larger defects with significant loss of both lamellae, advanced reconstructive techniques are necessary.

The surgeon's first choice of closure of large defects is usually to mobilize local tissue. In younger individuals with good skin tone and minimal skin and tendon laxity, little local tissue is available for mobilization. In older individuals, large defects may be closed with direct closure or development of small flaps.

The surgeon should assess the patient's skin tone and quality. Patients may have minimal skin available for flap formation if they have had prior surgery, trauma, or radiation treatment, or have certain dermatologic conditions.

Clinical Decision Making

Most simple skin lacerations can be repaired by direct closure. When possible, the direction of the incision or repair should be along the relaxed skin tension lines, to allow a less obvious scar. Care must be taken not to evert the eyelid margins when large horizontal wounds are closed.

Full-thickness eyelid lacerations can be repaired by direct closure. If the wound edges are irregular, they should be excised with scissors, and the wound prepared in a pentagonal wedge configuration. The edges can then be closed with the classic three-suture technique.

For lacerations to the canalicular system, the canaliculi should be inspected and intubated with Silastic tubing. When the tubing is placed under light tension, the wound edges move into close apposition. Although there is no tarsus present medial to the punctum, similar closure of the margin defect is performed with multiple superficial sutures, as well as absorbable sutures placed through the canthal tendon (Figure 6-1).

For a small defect (<25%) of an eyelid, direct closure is usually appropriate to bring wound edges together without placing excessive tension on the sutures. However in young patients, even a small defect may need to be repaired with the assistance of other methods. The surgeon can always assess the availability of tissue for direct closure by grasping the wound edges with forceps and gently drawing them together. If the edges can be apposed, then adequate tissue is present.

For most moderate (≤40%) eyelid defects in older adults, and for small defects in younger patients, the lateral wound edge may be mobilized by releasing the attachment of the lateral canthal tendon from the orbital rim. Lateral canthotomy involves incising the common crus of the canthal tendon, which provides a small amount of mobility to the lower eyelid. Inferior cantholysis releases the corresponding canthal tendon from its attachment to the orbital rim. Cantholysis is a "titratable" procedure. As more canthal fibers are incised, the eyelid gains significant mobility.

Defects that are too large to be closed by canthotomy and cantholysis may be closed with a lateral semicircular flap. This method is based on the concept of the canthotomy and cantholysis, but it additionally mobilizes skin lateral to the lateral canthus. The semicircular flap may be used to reconstruct defects up to 50% of the eyelid in adults.

In larger defects that cannot be closed by advancement of lateral tissue, typically following over 50% horizontal eyelid loss, tarsoconjunctival flaps may be created. For full-thickness upper eyelid deficits, a lower eyelid flap may be created from the lower lid. This procedure, known as a Cutler-Beard bridge flap, advances skin, muscle, and conjunctiva to the upper defect. To maintain stability of the upper lid, an autogenous cartilage graft may be placed anterior to the conjunctival layer.

For full-thickness lower eyelid reconstruction, a flap of tarsus and conjunctiva from the upper lid may provide adequate posterior lamella (Hughes procedure). Because the upper tarsus has approximately 10 mm vertical height, transfer of a small segment should not significantly alter the integrity of the eyelid. Skin may be advanced superiorly from the remaining lower eyelid or may be grafted from the upper lid or postauricular region.

Reconstruction of the medial canthal area is often complex because of the presence of the lacrimal drainage system. Medial canthal repair of large defects may require formation of a tarsoconjunc-

---

                                               Eyelid Reconstruction

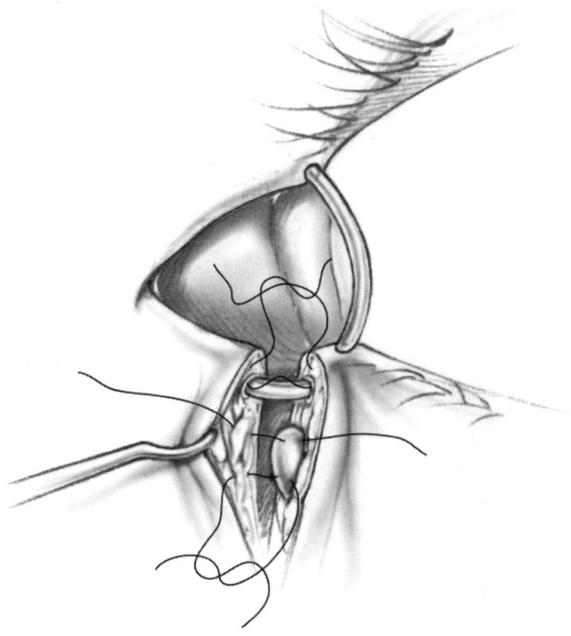

FIGURE 6-1. After the canalicular system has been intubated and before skin sutures are placed, the tendon and canaliculus are sutured.

tival flap from the upper eyelid, with a full-thickness graft to replace the skin deficit. Repair with a flap is often difficult because of the contour of the region and a lack of adequate skin that can be mobilized from surrounding areas. Contralateral upper eyelid skin or postauricular skin is usually the best match. When small medial canthal defects are present, the surgeon may choose to allow the region to heal by secondary intention. When proper wound care is followed, this area heals remarkably well. If an unacceptable scar results, the scar can be excised and reconstruction initiated.

MANAGEMENT

Medical Treatment Options

Prior to reconstruction, the wound should be kept moist with antibiotic ointment, and the cornea protected from exposure. Frequent application of lubricating drops or ointment to the ocular surface is recommended.

Some areas of the face heal well by secondary intention. These areas include the concave areas of the nose and ears, the temporal and glabellar regions, and the medial canthus. If a large defect is present, partial wound closure with "purse string" sutures may decrease healing time. The wound should be kept moist with antibiotic ointment until complete epithelialization has occurred, which may require several weeks or months. The wound should be cleaned twice a day to remove debris and crusting. If the healing by secondary intention is unfavorable, the process may be interrupted at any stage and reconstruction initiated.

Surgical Treatment Options

Most surgical procedures are performed in the operating room under intravenous sedation. Local anesthetic, 2% lidocaine with epinephrine, is provided subcutaneously. Appropriate sterile prep and drape is performed for all patients.

Pentagonal Resection of an Eyelid Tumor, with Direct Closure

Direct closure of small full-thickness eyelid wounds following mass excision can commonly be performed in patients who have moderate or marked eyelid laxity. The same classic three-suture technique should also be performed for full-thickness eyelid lacerations involving the margin when there is no significant tissue loss. This method provides secure wound closure and eversion of the eyelid margin, allowing the edge to reform its smooth contour. During the initial repair, the wound edges should be converted into a pentagonal configuration by excising the irregular edges.

Prior to excision of a margin mass, the borders of the lesion are marked. If a malignancy is suspected, appropriate borders of normal-appearing skin are included in the resection (Figure 6-2). A #11 blade is used to create the vertical incisions through the margin. The incisions are initiated along the inferior aspect of the vertical markings and advanced through the entire eyelid, with attention to the globe, to avoid damaging it. The blade is advanced superiorly through the margin, to create a smooth wound edge. If the entire vertical arm of the incision is not completed, the blade may be reversed and the cut extended inferiorly to the appropriate level. Westcott scissors are used to complete the pentagonal incision.

Margin repair involves passing three 6-0 silk sutures through corresponding points on both sides of the wound (Figure 6-3). The clas-

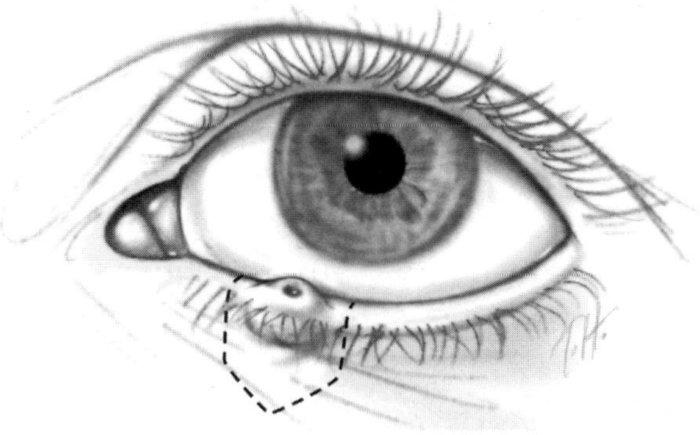

FIGURE 6-2. The mass is outlined with appropriate margins in the form of a pentagon.

sic landmarks are the lash line (anterior suture), meibomian gland orifices (middle), and mucocutaneous junction (posterior). Sutures do not need to be placed precisely through these landmarks, but they should be evenly spaced and should contain equal amount of tissue on each side of the wound. The surgeon should not place the posterior suture in a position where it can abrade the conjunctiva or cornea.

The sutures are placed 1–2 mm from the lacerated wound edge to a depth that equals the distance from the wound edge. The sutures are not tied immediately. The surgeon should confirm that equal amounts of tissue at corresponding levels are involved. The surgeon

FIGURE 6-3. Several 6-0 silk sutures are placed at the eyelid margin and a 5-0 Vicryl suture is placed through the tarsus.

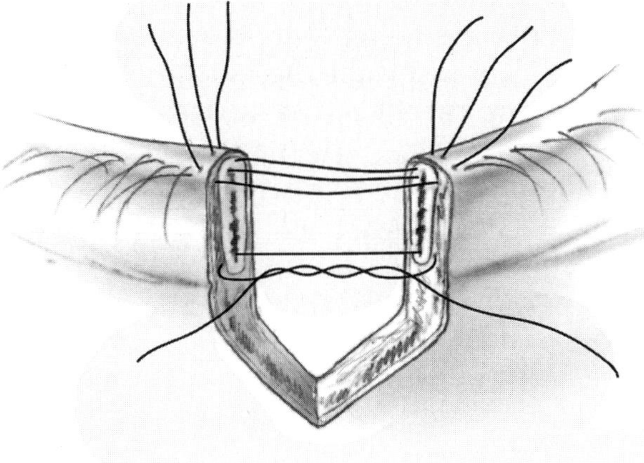

or an assistant can cross both ends of the most anterior suture to bring the margin together, verifying that the edges move into good position and that the wound will not be under excessive tension. If the margin is not properly aligned, the suture should be removed and passed again. If excessive tension persists, other reconstructive techniques should be implemented.

The surgeon can tie the middle suture to verify that the wounds are under minimal tension and have appropriate alignment. After all three margin sutures are secured, the needles are removed but the tails are left long. The tails are placed on light tension to expose the remainder of the wound.

The tarsus is closed with one or two simple interrupted 5-0 or 6-0 Vicryl sutures, placed in the partial-thickness manner to avoid irritation to the cornea. For upper eyelid wounds, an additional suture may be used to stabilize the larger tarsus. These tarsal sutures generally provide adequate deep tissue support for the entire wound, and additional deep sutures are not necessary. The eyelid margin should be slightly everted at this point. During the healing phase, as the scar contracts, the margin will become even. Several optional subcutaneous Vicryl sutures may be placed to provide additional support for skin closure.

The skin is closed with running or interrupted 6-0 plain gut sutures. The tails of the margin silk sutures are tied over the skin with a 6-0 silk suture, placed several millimeters from the lash line, to prevent abrasion of the eye (Figure 6-4). When the margin sutures are secure, the tails of the remaining sutures are cut. The sutures are removed in 10–14 days.

Canthotomy and Cantholysis

When a significant part of the eyelid (approximately one-third) is absent and direct closure is not possible, additional horizontal lengthening is commonly performed. This situation frequently occurs following removal of medium-sized tumors of the lower eyelid. One commonly performed option of mobilizing the tissue necessary for wound closure involves canthotomy and cantholysis. In these steps, the lateral canthus is incised (canthotomy) and the upper or lower crus partially or completely released (cantholysis) from the periosteum of the orbital rim.

Curved Stevens scissors are used to incise the lateral canthus to the orbital rim, completing the lateral canthotomy (Figure 6-5). Many surgeons prefer to initially "crush" the lateral canthus with a hemostat, which is placed horizontally at the lateral canthal angle with

Eyelid Reconstruction

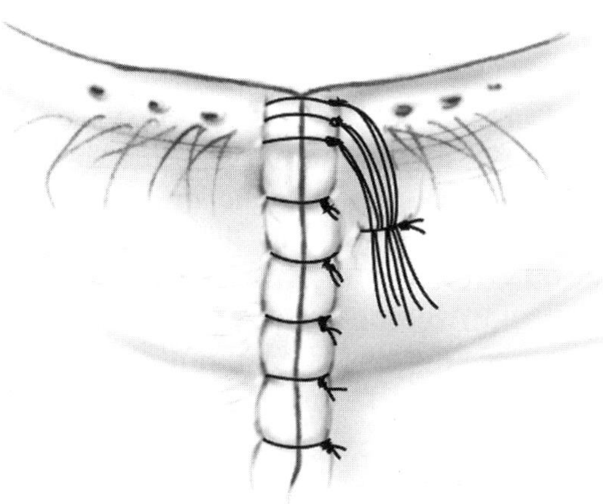

FIGURE 6-4. Eyelid margin sutures are tied to the skin to prevent abrasion of the eye. Skin sutures are placed.

one of the instrument blades on the conjunctival surface and one on skin. The hemostat is advanced posteriorly until the lateral orbital rim is palpated and then is tightened for several seconds to compress the canthus. This maneuver may assist in hemostasis and allow an even incision along the tissue. However, this step is not necessary.

While the canthotomy may provide several millimeters of horizontal laxity, it usually needs to be followed by cantholysis to provide adequate horizontal tissue mobility and to allow closure of lower eyelid defects. The lateral margin edge of the defect is then grasped with forceps or a small skin hook and pulled toward the opposite

FIGURE 6-5. A lateral canthotomy is completed with scissors.

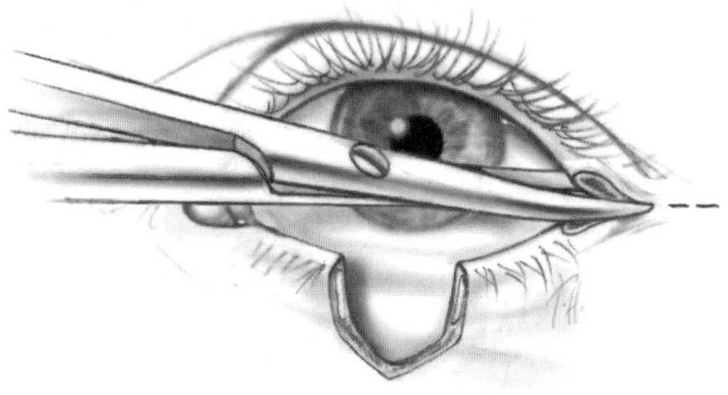

wound edge. If the edges are not in apposition, cantholysis should be performed.

The lateral portion of the eyelid can be grasped with forceps several millimeters from the canthotomy incision, and the lid gently stretched outward and medially, to place tension on the inferior limb of the lateral canthal tendon. With Westcott scissors placed through the canthotomy incision, the surgeon can palpate the canthal tendon between skin and conjunctiva. As small incisions are made through the tendon, the eyelid becomes more mobile, and the defect can be closed. After each incision of the tendon, the edges of the wound should be grasped with toothed forceps and the amount of overlap and tension of the defect tested. This portion of the operation is titratable, and often it is not necessary to incise the entire tendon (Figure 6-6).

As with direct closure, approximately 2 mm of overlap with minimal or no tension is recommended. The margin defect is closed as a pentagonal wedge with the standard three-suture technique. Three simple interrupted 6-0 silk sutures are preplaced in the eyelid margin. One suture is placed along the eyelash margin. A second suture is placed in the central eyelid margin, typically at the meibomian gland orifices. The final suture is placed along the posterior eyelid margin, at the mucocutaneous junction, with particular attention to avoiding contact between the tied suture and the eye.

To reduce tension on the wound, an assistant crosses the central suture. The anterior suture is tied first; then the other two margin sutures are secured. One or two interrupted 6-0 Vicryl sutures are placed through the tarsus in a partial-thickness manner. These sutures are important to stabilize the wound. The surgeon should not place these sutures through the conjunctiva, where they would cause irritation to the eye. Additional subcutaneous inverted interrupted 6-0 Vicryl sutures may be placed through the orbicularis muscle to reduce skin tension and improve apposition. Skin closure is accomplished with interrupted or running 6-0 plain gut suture.

To prevent the silk margin sutures from abrading the cornea, an interrupted 6-0 silk suture is placed below the eyelid margin and tied loosely to the skin. The ends of the margin sutures are gently stretched inferiorly and tied into this retaining suture. The suture ends are cut.

The new lateral canthal angle is re-formed with a simple interrupted 6-0 plain gut suture (Figure 6-7). This suture is placed through the lateral edge of the upper eyelid margin, at the site of the previous lateral canthal angle. The suture is next placed through the conjunctiva and then through the skin of the lateral edge of the lower

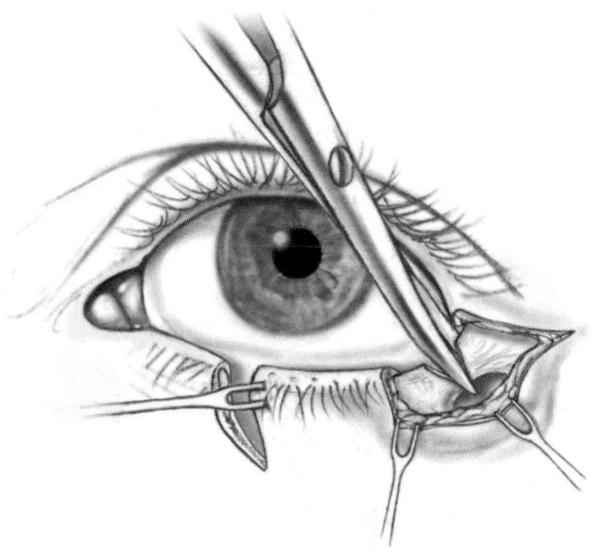

FIGURE 6-6. A cantholysis is performed by stretching the eyelid medially and incising the corresponding canthal tendon.

FIGURE 6-7. The eyelid defect is closed with a classic three-suture technique. The lateral canthal angle is reformed, and the skin edges are closed. Suturing conjunctiva to the skin edge reforms the lateral eyelid margin.

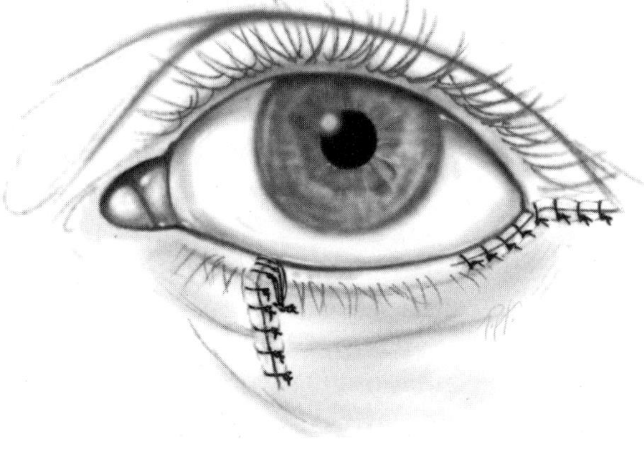

eyelid. When the suture is tied, the new lateral canthal angle is formed. Additional interrupted or running 6-0 plain gut sutures are placed to close the remaining lateral skin incision.

The reconstructed portion of the lower eyelid margin is reformed. One or more buried 6-0 plain gut sutures are placed through the skin edge and then through the conjunctival edge, and tied. These sutures allow the conjunctiva to cover the rough skin at the new lid margin and reduce the risk of abrasion to the eye. The silk sutures are removed in 10–14 days.

"Tenzel" Semicircular Advancement Flap

The semicircular temporal advancement flap allows the surgeon to mobilize a larger amount of tissue lateral to the defect than is possible with the canthotomy and cantholysis procedure. The semicircular advancement flap procedure is particularly useful when both sides of the wound contain tarsus. The incision begins at the lateral canthus and extends temporally in a semicircular manner. As the flap is rotated and closed, the wound flattens to correspond to the facial lines.

A semicircular temporal advancement flap is frequently developed following excision of lower eyelid neoplasms. Standard mass excision includes marking the borders with appropriate margins. The vertical incisions are created with a #11 blade, passed full thickness through the edges of the wound. The blade is advanced superiorly, through the margin, to create smooth, even wound edges. Westcott scissors are used to complete the removal of the lesion. The specimen is marked with suture to clarify the proper orientation, and the specimen is sent to the pathology department for review.

When the surgeon is ready to reconstruct the eyelid, the edges of the tissue are gently advanced together with forceps, to estimate the sizes of the defect and to determine whether additional tissue needs to be mobilized for closure. The wound should be trimmed to form a pentagon before a Tenzel flap is mobilized.

A curved line is marked on the skin beginning at the lateral canthus. For lower eyelid flaps, the incision should arch superiorly; and for upper eyelid flaps, the incision should arch inferiorly (Figure 6-8). A typical flap extends two-thirds of the distance from the canthus to the hairline, but larger flaps may be created. A #15 blade is used to develop the incision through skin and muscle. The plane beneath orbicularis is dissected with scissors to mobilize the entire flap.

A lateral canthotomy is performed through the initial incision. The lower lid can be mobilized with cantholysis (Figure 6-9). These maneuvers should provide significant mobility to the eyelid. If the

Eyelid Reconstruction

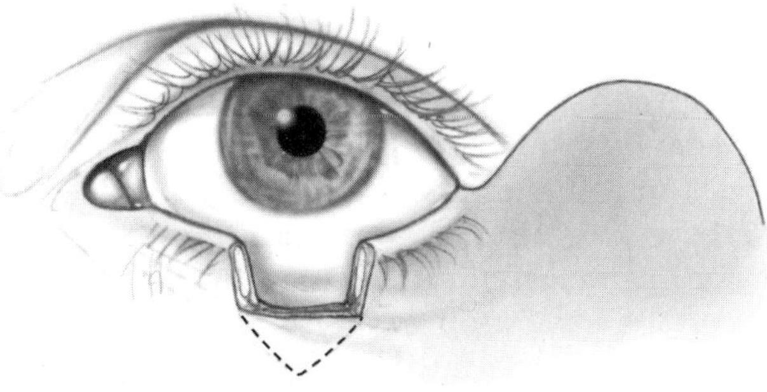

FIGURE 6-8. A large eyelid defect is trimmed to form a pentagon. The lateral canthal incision is marked.

wound edges still cannot be brought into apposition, further undermining of the flap may be performed to allow maximal rotation of the flap. When the wound edges can be apposed without tension, the three-suture technique is utilized for closure.

The standard eyelid margin closure utilizes three 6-0 silk margin sutures. These sutures are placed at the posterior eyelid margin, the meibomian gland orifices, and at the posterior edge of the lash line. An assistant crosses one of the margin sutures to bring to eyelid into proper position, allowing the surgeon to tie the other margin sutures without significant wound tension. If the margin appears to have good contour, the final silk suture is tied. The ends of the sutures should

FIGURE 6-9. A skin-orbicularis flap is elevated. A lateral canthotomy and cantholysis are completed, and the eyelid is mobilized.

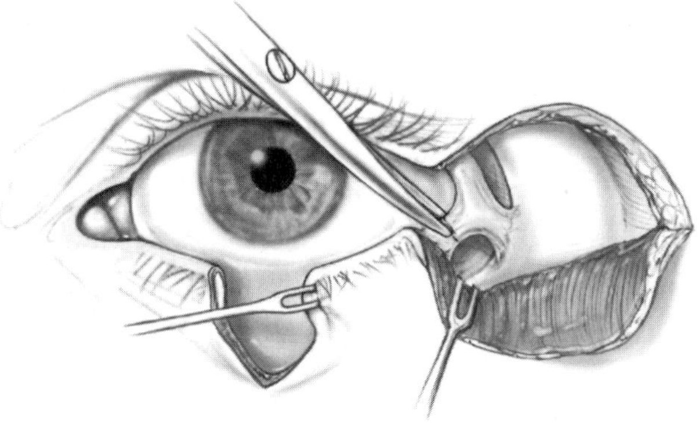

not be cut at this time; rather, they should be used to place gentle superior retraction during the remaining closure of the margin.

One or two simple interrupted 6-0 Vicryl sutures are placed in a partial-thickness manner through tarsus, and tied. Several simple interrupted subcutaneous inverted 6-0 Vicryl sutures are placed to reduce tension on the skin edges. Running or simple interrupted 6-0 plain gut sutures are used for skin closure. A simple interrupted 6-0 silk suture is tied loosely over the skin, approximately 5–7 mm from the margin. The ends of the silk margin sutures are rotated inferiorly and tied to the recently placed silk skin suture, to prevent the margin sutures from irritating the globe.

The new lateral canthal angle is formed by passing a 6-0 Vicryl suture from the skin edge, through a lateral remnant of palpebral conjunctiva, and through the lateral edge of the normal upper eyelid (Figure 6-10). The posterior aspect of the newly rotated advancement flap is composed of muscular tissue. The underlying conjunctiva should be undermined and advanced to the edge of the flap to form a new margin. The new eyelid margin is formed by passing several buried simple interrupted 6-0 plain gut sutures from the skin edge through the remaining palpebral conjunctiva. Mucous membrane grafting using a free conjunctival or buccal mucosal graft is an alternative means preparing the posterior surface or the flap.

To prevent retraction of the newly reconstructed eyelid, a 5-0 Vicryl suture is passed from subcutaneous tissue of the flap to the periosteum of the lateral orbital rim. When this suture is tied, mild over correction of the eyelid should exist. Several inverted simple interrupted 6-0 Vicryl sutures are placed in the subcutaneous plane of the skin, and the skin edges are closed with running or multiple interrupted 6-0 plain gut sutures (Figure 6-11).

Upper Eyelid Tarsoconjunctival Reconstruction (Cutler-Beard)

The "Cutler-Beard" bridge flap is useful for reconstructing large upper eyelid defects, particularly those that are located centrally. The upper wound edges are trimmed and made perpendicular to the margin, and the lower eyelid flap is developed.

The lower eyelid skin is carefully marked, beginning 3.5 mm inferior to the margin, to avoid incising the marginal arterial arcade (Figure 6-12). A corresponding mark is made on the conjunctival side of the eyelid. The horizontal length of the flap should equal the width of the upper defect. At the ends of the skin marking, vertical lines can be extended inferiorly.

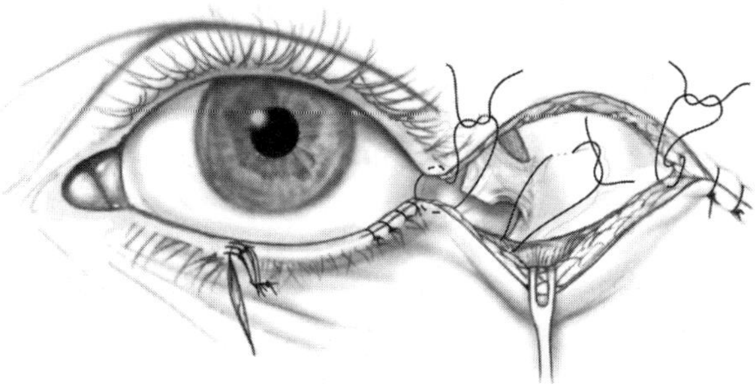

FIGURE 6-10. The defect is closed with the classic three-suture technique. The lateral canthal angle is recreated, and joining the edges of conjunctiva and skin re-forms the lateral eyelid margin. The orbicularis is secured to the periosteum.

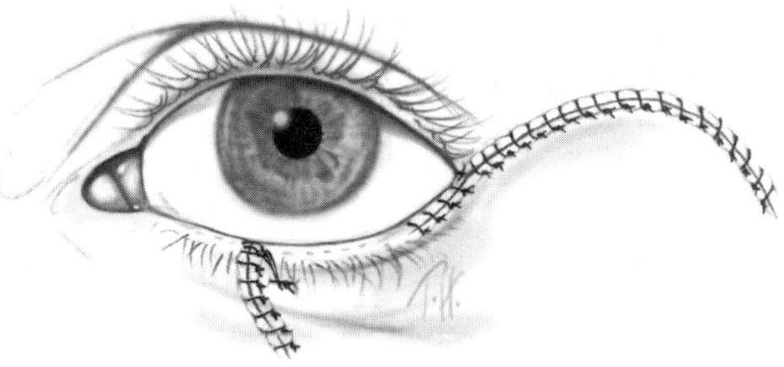

FIGURE 6-11. Skin sutures are placed, closing both wounds.

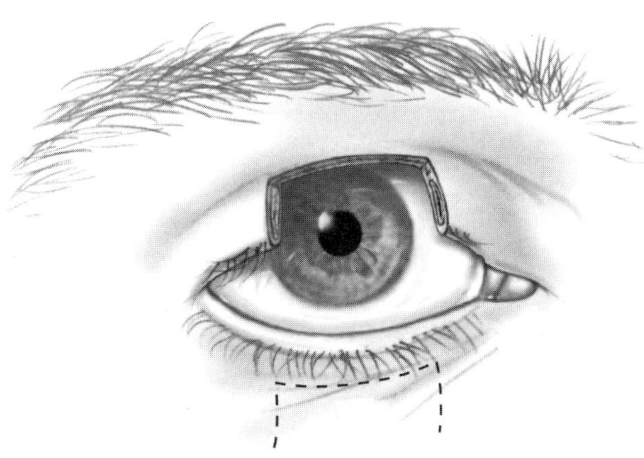

FIGURE 6-12. A large central upper eyelid defect is trimmed and a lower eyelid bridge flap is outlined to the same width.

The incision through skin and orbicularis is made with a blade. The eyelid is everted, and the same blade is used to make a corresponding incision through the conjunctiva and tarsus. The two incisions are joined with sharp Westcott scissors. This process of making two incisions helps the surgeon to avoid damaging the marginal arcade. With the same scissors, the full-thickness incision can be extended horizontally in both directions to the predetermined edges of the flap. The surgeon must remember to remain 3.5 mm from the margin at all times during the incision.

The lower eyelid bridge that is developed is important in retaining the normal appearance and function of the reconstructed lower eyelid. During the remainder of the procedure, a small Penrose drain is used to hold the bridge out of the surgical field with light traction.

At the ends of the horizontal incisions, vertical full-thickness incisions are made inferiorly, forming a lower eyelid advancement flap. This flap is gently placed under the lower eyelid bridge and then placed into the upper eyelid defect. The flap must fill the defect and have no significant inferior traction. Additional lower eyelid tissue may be advanced by extending the vertical incisions along the flap edge.

The conjunctiva of the upper edge of the wound is gently pulled inferiorly with forceps. The skin edge may be retracted superiorly by the assistant. Upon separating the tissue plains, the white edge of the levator can be identified above the conjunctiva.

Three layers of closure are recommended for this procedure. The upper eyelid conjunctiva is connected by multiple interrupted 6-0 plain gut sutures to the conjunctiva of the bridge flap (Figure 6-13). Some surgeons may elect to place a cartilage graft to provide additional stability to the eyelid. If a graft will be placed, the lower eyelid conjunctiva should be gently separated from the overlying tissue for several millimeters, to serve as a recipient site for the cartilage graft. Ear cartilage graft (or other suitable material) is harvested, trimmed, and secured to the levator (superiorly) and tarsus (sides) with 6-0 Vicryl interrupted sutures. The skin-orbicularis layer is closed with interrupted 6-0 plain gut suture.

If a graft is not performed, two additional layers of closure are planned. The middle layer of closure involves joining the remnant of the levator aponeurosis to the orbicularis muscle or the bridge flap. The superficial closure involves closing the skin.

The middle layer is closed with multiple interrupted 7-0 Vicryl sutures, connecting the orbicularis of the bridge flap to the levator aponeurosis at the upper aspect of the defect. This closure is important to ensure good movement of the reconstructed upper eyelid.

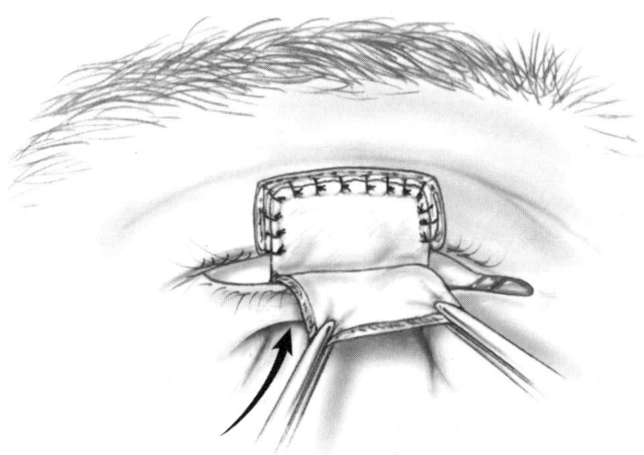

FIGURE 6-13. The conjunctival layer may be closed with interrupted 6-0 plain gut sutures. The levator may be sutured to the orbicularis layer, or a cartilage graft may be placed over conjunctiva and secured to the tarsus and levator.

The skin is closed with multiple interrupted 6-0 plain gut sutures (Figure 6-14). The surgeon should also pay attention to closure of the skin edges along the upper eyelid margin. The skin closure along the inferior portion of the advancement flap to the lower eyelid is completed at the medial and lateral edges. Direct closure of additional wounds that extend into the canthal regions should be performed with 6-0 plain gut suture.

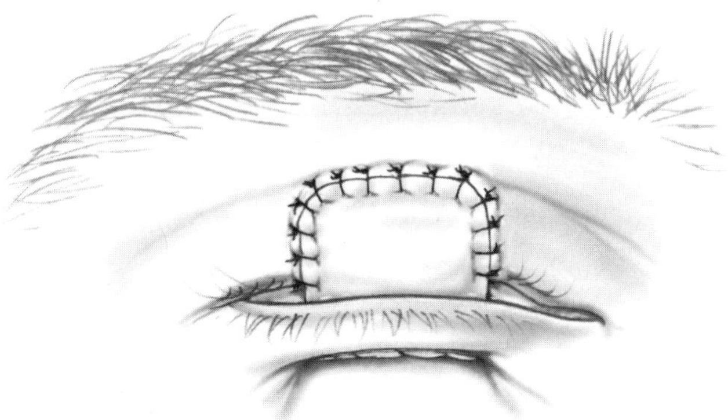

FIGURE 6-14. Skin closure is completed with interrupted sutures.

The entire completed bridge flap can be inspected under the bridge of normal eyelid tissue. A pressure dressing or bolster should be avoided, to ensure that the flap circulation is not compromised. The flap can be severed along the palpebral fissure and the eyelids reconstructed after approximately 3 weeks. The inferior margin of the bridge should be denuded with a blade or scissors and sutured to the upper margin of the skin flap with absorbable sutures (Figure 6-15). The upper eyelid may be sculpted with thermal cautery; the margin will re-epithelialize within several days.

Lower Eyelid Tarsoconjunctival Reconstruction (Hughes)

The Hughes tarsoconjunctival flap can be used to replace the posterior lamella in large lower eyelid reconstructions. The flap may be secured at its lateral and medial borders to existing lower eyelid tarsus or to a periosteal flap at the canthus. The tarsal flap is then covered by a skin flap or graft.

The lower eyelid tumor is identified, and several millimeters of normal-appearing tissue are marked. The skin is incised with a blade, and the tumor is removed with scissors. The lower lid wound edges are made perpendicular to the margin. If permanent section analysis of the margins is desired, thin tissue specimens, taken from the medial, lateral, and inferior borders of the defect, are sent to the pathology department for further analysis.

Temporary eyelid closure can be performed to protect the cornea and stretch the remaining eyelid skin, to prevent contraction. A 4-0 silk mattress suture is passed through the temporal portion of the remaining eyelid, then through the inferior and medial portions of the lid. The suture is tied over cotton bolsters. Once complete tumor removal has been confirmed, the mattress suture is removed.

The edges of the wound are debrided with a blade. The size of the defect is measured. The width of the upper eyelid flap should be at least 2 mm wider than the defect, so the ends can be positioned into the lower eyelid "grooves." The upper eyelid is marked on the tarsal surface. The surgeon must leave at least 3.5 mm of tarsus on the upper eyelid, to allow proper stability.

A blade is used to make an incision through conjunctiva and tarsus (Figure 6-16). Westcott scissors are used to dissect the tarsus from the overlying orbicularis. Once the tarsus is free, the surgical plane continues superiorly, just above the conjunctiva. To improve exposure, the surgeon gently pulls the tarsus inferiorly, and an assistant

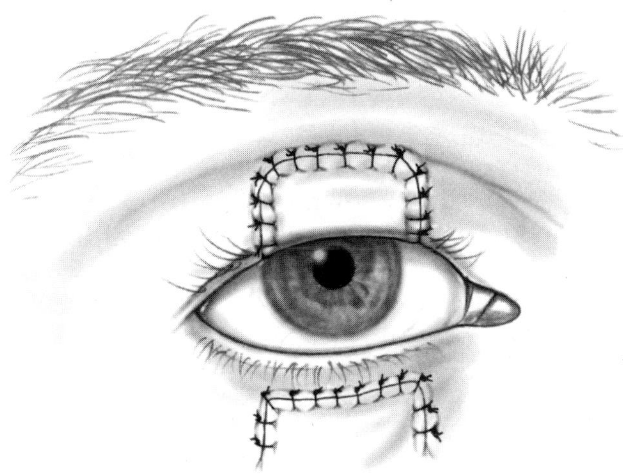

FIGURE 6-15. After the bridge flap has been severed, it is reattached to the lower eyelid margin.

lifts the skin-muscle plane superiorly. The surgeon should be able to visualize the tips of the scissors through the conjunctiva at all times.

Vertical incisions along the lateral and medial edges of the conjunctival flap are made, to form a flap that will correspond to the lower eyelid defect. The flap should be positioned in the lower eyelid

FIGURE 6-16. A tarsoconjunctival flap is incised and dissected from upper eyelid to correspond in width to the width of the defect. It is sutured to the lower eyelid conjunctiva. A lower eyelid advancement flap is marked.

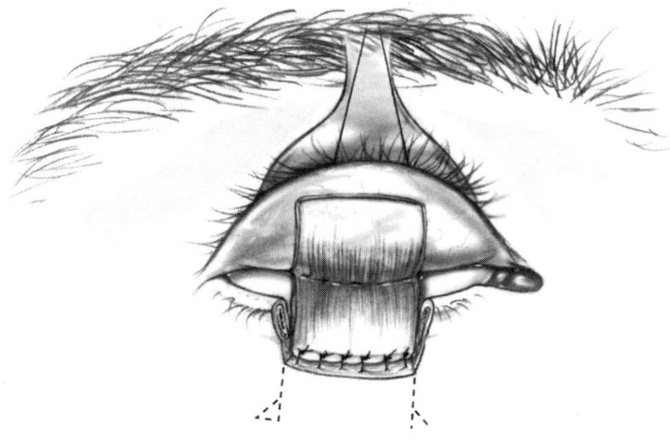

deficit. If upward traction persists, additional conjunctival dissection and extended lateral incisions should be performed. The inferior tarsal border of the flap is secured to the remaining conjunctiva of the lower eyelid defect with interrupted 6-0 Vicryl sutures.

The recipient eyelid is "grooved" by splitting the anterior and posterior lamellae for 2–3 mm with scissors, allowing the medial and lateral ends of the tarsoconjunctival flap to be secured to the remnants of the lower eyelid (Figure 6-17). A double-armed 6-0 silk mattress suture is used to secure the flap within the "grooved" lower eyelid. The ends of the 6-0 silk suture are passed through the lower lid conjunctiva and tarsus (or periosteal flap) and into the "groove." The needles are passed through the ends of the flap and out through the skin, several millimeters from the edge of the wound. The sutures are tied over a small rubber band. The tarsoconjunctival flap is secured in this manner on its lateral and medial ends. At this point, the flap has been secured on three sides. The tarsus from the upper eyelid can be seen to align with the remaining tarsus of the lower eyelid.

The tarsal flap can be covered with a sliding advancement skin flap developed from the eyelid and cheek inferior to the wound (Figure 6-18). Vertical incisions can be made inferiorly, from the vertical edges of the wound defect. The skin flap should not place inferior tension on the wound. Also, to reduce the chance of postoperative retraction, the flap should not incorporate muscle.

The superior aspect of the skin flap is tied to the upper aspect of the donor tarsus with multiple interrupted 6-0 plain gut sutures. The lateral edge of the skin flap must be correctly attached to the skin of the remaining eyelid margin with an interrupted 6-0 silk suture. A similar suture is placed medially to connect the skin flap to the medial eyelid margin remnant. The remaining skin edges can be closed with interrupted 6-0 plain gut sutures. Alternatively a full-thickness skin graft can be prepared and secured.

The conjunctival bridge may be severed in 3–6 weeks (Figure 6-19). The new lid margin may be sculpted with thermal cautery if any surface irregularities persist.

Medial Canthal Tumor Excision with Retroauricular Skin Graft

Closure of small medial canthal defects can usually be performed directly, or the areas can be allowed to granulate. The concavity of the region, and proximity to the eyelids and brow, are factors that limit the development of flaps for closure of larger defects. Skin grafts

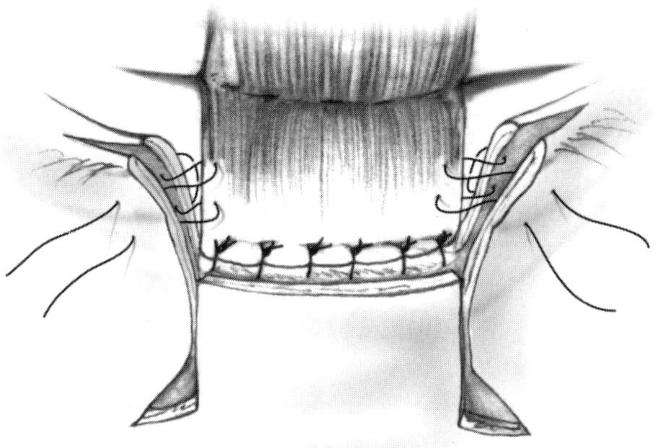

FIGURE 6-17. Lower eyelid grooves are created to secure the position of the upper tarsus.

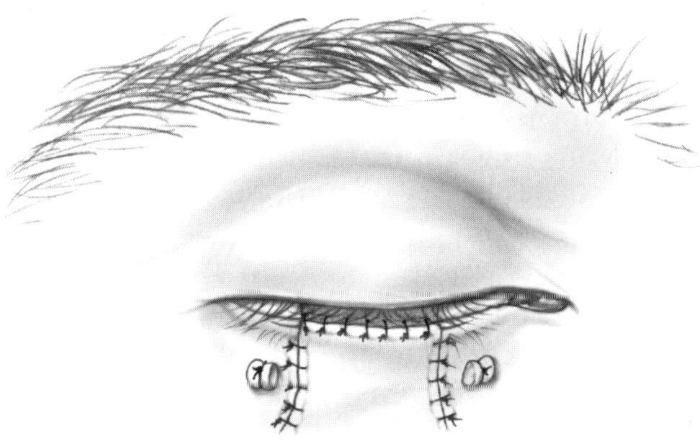

FIGURE 6-18. A lower eyelid sliding advancement flap is mobilized and sutured to the skin edges. This covers the upper eyelid flap.

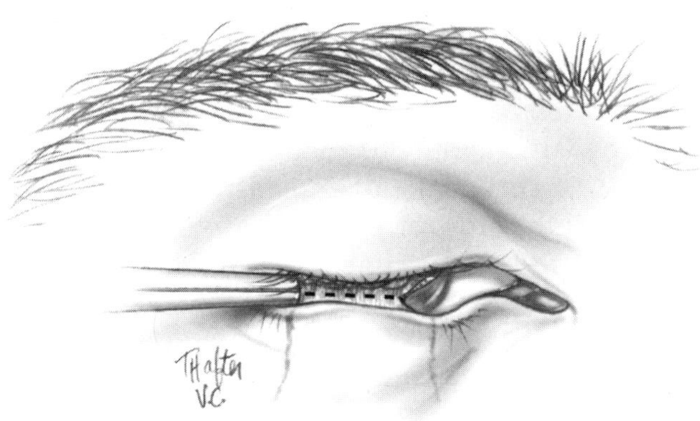

FIGURE 6-19. In several weeks, the bridge is severed with scissors. A smooth, blunt instrument is placed behind the scissors to protect the eye.

tend to provide adequate coverage and heal well for reconstruction of most medial canthal defects.

At the beginning of the procedure, the donor retroauricular site is injected with approximately 2 mL of 2% lidocaine with epinephrine in the subcutaneous plane. The injection should manually elevate the skin, to provide easy dissection later. A small amount of infiltrate is also provided about 1 cm anterior to the helix, where the traction suture will be placed.

To excise a medial canthal mass, the surgeon first delineates the suspected location with a marking pen, allowing several millimeters of normal skin surrounding a suspected malignancy (Figure 6-20). The specimen can be marked with suture to provide correct orientation and is sent for frozen section analysis. The depth of the dissection should be at least through the orbicularis muscle. Thorough hemostasis is mandatory.

When a retroauricular skin graft is planned, a traction suture should be placed to hold the ear in position. A 4-0 silk mattress suture, placed through the skin over the outer aspect of the helix and the preauricular skin, is tied securely. This suture places the retroauricular skin in tension and provides excellent visualization.

A piece of Telfa is cut with scissors to match the size and shape of the medial canthal defect. This material will serve as a template for the graft. The template is placed over the donor site and outlined with a marking pen. The donor skin should be approximately 25% larger than the defect, because graft contraction will occur as the tissue heals. To facilitate closure, "wings" may be added to the outline along the crease of the sulcus, forming an ellipse (Figure 6-21). The ellipse is excised with a #15 blade and Westcott scissors. The surgeon should be careful to remove a thin graft, with little subcutaneous tissue. Excessive subcutaneous tissue will lessen the chances for a successful graft.

Following removal of the graft, further thinning is performed. The graft must be handled with extreme care. The graft can be placed flat on the surgeon's gloved finger, with the subcutaneous side facing up. Westcott scissors, held parallel to the graft, are used to trim excess subcutaneous tissue from the underside of the tissue. If the graft begins to move or "bunch up," it should be placed flat again against the finger before more subcutaneous tissue is removed. If the graft is not resting flat, the scissors may penetrate the surface and create a "buttonhole."

Multiple interrupted 6-0 plain gut sutures are used to secure the graft to the wound edges. Antibiotic ointment may be placed over the

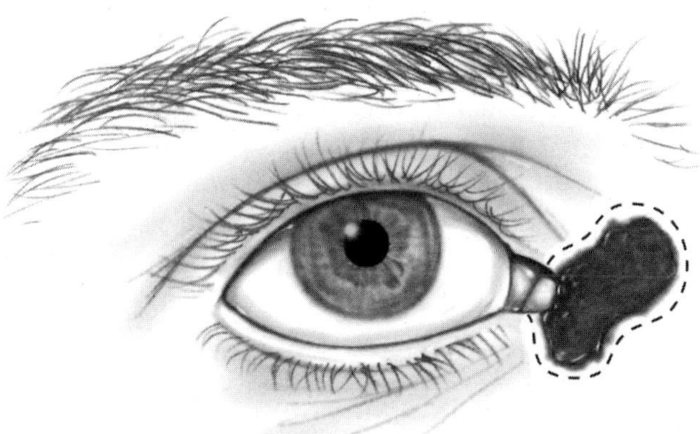

FIGURE 6-20. A medial canthal tumor is marked with appropriate borders and excised.

FIGURE 6-21. A full-thickness skin graft can be harvested from the retroauricular sulcus.

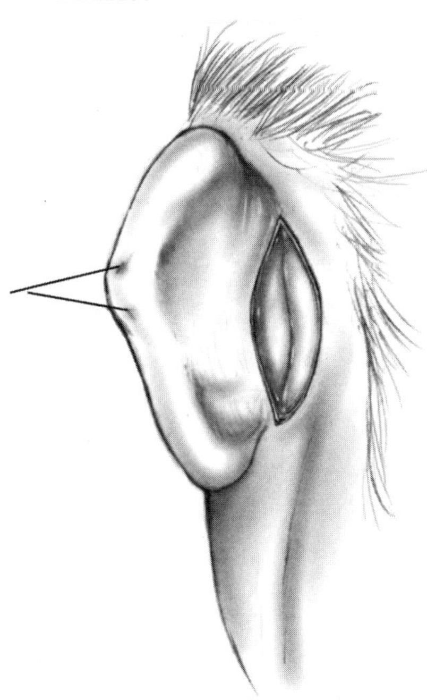

wound. Several 6-0 silk or nylon sutures are placed several millimeters away from the graft edge. The ends of these permanent sutures are left long, because they will be used to tie a cotton-Telfa bolster over the graft (Figure 6-22). A small bolster may be held securely with only two sutures, but larger bolsters may require up to eight sutures. A small piece of Telfa is placed over the graft and covered by a wet piece of cotton. The permanent sutures are tied over the cotton; they will hold light pressure on the graft for the first postoperative week (Figure 6-23).

After meticulous hemostasis has been achieved, the retroauricular lesion is closed with 5-0 chromic sutures, placed in a near-far-far-near or other tension-reducing pattern. The wound is covered with antibiotic ointment, and a Glasscock-type dressing is placed on the ear. This dressing places mild tension on the ear, to reduce the incidence of postoperative bleeding.

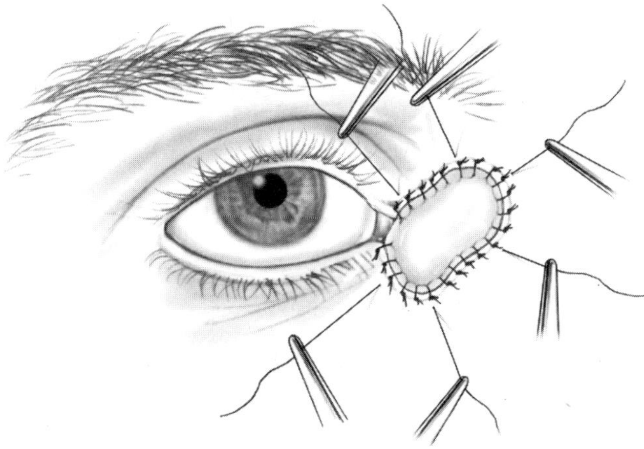

FIGURE 6-22. A skin graft is sutured over the wound. Multiple 6-0 silk sutures, placed several millimeters from graft, will be used to secure the bolster.

FIGURE 6-23. A bolster is secured over the skin graft.

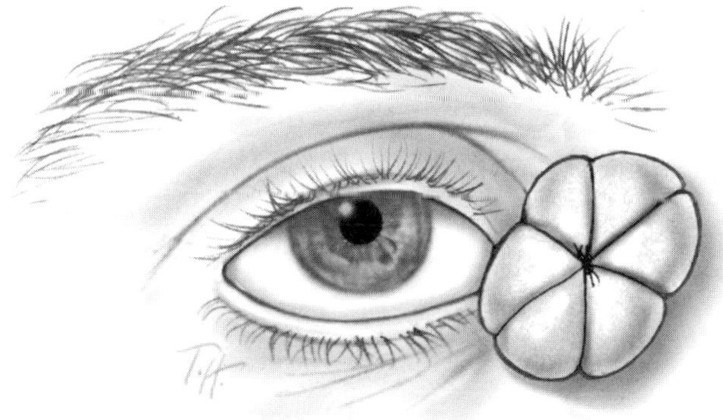

INDEX

ISBN 0-387-95316-7

Contributors

GEOFFREY J. GLADSTONE

EVAN H. BLACK

SHOIB MYINT

BRIAN G. BRAZZO

FRANK A. NESI

BRIGGS E. COOK

BRADLEY N. LEMKE

MARK J. LUCARELLI

JOHN G. ROSE, JR.

Contents